PRAISE FOR
VOLUNTEERING AT HOME AND ABROAD:
THE ESSENTIAL GUIDE FOR NURSES

"Most nurses are fortunate to have wealth in knowledge, skills, expertise, health, and family, and sufficient resources for a quality life. When we work with others who do not have these gifts, it challenges us to think about how wasteful we can be and how fortunate we are. Enjoy reading this guide and planning for an adventure that will change your life."

–William L. Holzemer, PhD, RN, FAAN
Dean and Professor, Rutgers University
Member, Board of Directors, International Council of Nurses

"If you are looking for a comprehensive and unique contribution to the literature on global health volunteering in nursing, this is the text for you! It is perhaps the most thorough coverage of volunteering in nursing from the early history of Florence Nightingale to present-day volunteering in disaster relief and resource-limited settings. It is a must-have for those who are considering volunteering nationally and internationally."

–Patrice K. Nicholas, DNSc, RN, ANP, FAAN
Director of Global Health and Academic Partnerships, Brigham and Women's Hospital
Division of Global Health Equity and Center for Nursing Excellence
Professor, MGH Institute of Health Professions School of Nursing
Director, Honor Society of Nursing, Sigma Theta Tau International

"This is a must-read for nurses seeking global health volunteer experiences. It is a contemporary, practical guide that addresses the multitude of questions ranging from 'Where can I go?' to 'How can I be culturally and politically sensitive when I get there?' As a faculty member working with a whole host of students searching for global health experiences, it is a much-needed and welcome reference."

–Sara Groves, DrPH, APRN-BC
The Johns Hopkins University School of Nursing
Gates Grant Liaison in Uganda

"As a nurse educator who has volunteered in developing countries for more than 14 years, I am thrilled to see this book. Jeanne Leffers, Julia Plotnick, and their contributors cover the essential components of volunteering in an easy-to-read book that will serve as a guide to any nurse who is considering volunteering in any setting. This is the most thorough resource that is available for nurse volunteers and is a must-read for new and seasoned volunteers."

–Jill B. Derstine, EdD, RN, FAAN
Professor Emerita, Temple University
Clinical Associate Professor, Drexel University

"I share the authors' perspectives that nurses should spend time assessing their strengths and limitations as a volunteer, preparing themselves well in advance for this important nursing role, and working with an established volunteer agency. The authors' personal experiences provide helpful insight into and guidance for how to prepare to be an effective nurse volunteer. The tools for self-assessment and matching one's expertise to the needs of the volunteer agency lead the reader to consider key personal, practical, and ethical aspects of volunteering, especially in cultures other than one's own."

–Joyce E. Thompson, DrPH, RN, CNM, FAAN, FACNM
International Consultant in Women's Health, Midwifery, Nursing, & Health Care Ethics
Professor Emerita, University of Pennsylvania and Western Michigan University

VOLUNTEERING
AT HOME AND ABROAD:
THE ESSENTIAL GUIDE
FOR NURSES

Jeanne Leffers, PhD, RN
Julia Plotnick, MPH, RN, FAAN

Sigma Theta Tau International
Honor Society of Nursing®

Sigma Theta Tau International

The Honor Society of Nursing, Sigma Theta Tau International, the only international honor society worldwide, is a global community of nurse leaders with members who live in 86 countries and belong to 469 chapters. Through this network, members lead in using knowledge, scholarship, service, and learning to improve the health of the world's people.

Sigma Theta Tau International
550 West North Street
Indianapolis, IN 46202

To order additional books, buy in bulk, or order for corporate use, contact Nursing Knowledge International TOLL FREE at 888.654.4968 (US and Canada) or +1.317.634.8171 (outside US and Canada).

To request a review copy for course adoption, e-mail solutions@nursingknowledge.org or call TOLL FREE at 888.654.4968 (US and Canada) or +1.317.634.8171 (outside US and Canada).

To request author information, or for speaker or other media requests, contact Rachael McLaughlin of the Honor Society of Nursing, Sigma Theta Tau International at 888.634.7575 (US and Canada) or +1.317.634.8171 (outside US and Canada).

ISBN-13:   9781-930538-98-6
EPUB and Mobi ISBN: 9781-935476-382
PDF ISBN: 9781-935476-399

Library of Congress Cataloging-in-Publication Data

Leffers, Jeanne, 1947-
  Volunteering at home and abroad : the essential guide for nurses / Jeanne Leffers, Julia Plotnick.
     p. ; cm.
  Includes bibliographical references and index.
  ISBN 978-1-930538-98-6 (alk. paper)
  1. Nursing. 2. Volunteer workers in medical care. I. Plotnick, Julia, 1936- II. Sigma Theta Tau International. III. Title.
  [DNLM: 1. Nurses. 2. Voluntary Programs. 3. Voluntary Workers. WY 16.1]
  RT82.L34 2011
  362.17'3--dc22
                        2011012692

First Printing, 2011

Publisher: Renee Wilmeth
Acquisitions Editor: Janet Boivin, RN
Editorial Coordinator: Paula Jeffers
Proofreaders: Barbara Bennett and Jane Palmer
Cover Design: Katy Bodenmiller

Development Editor: Carla Hall
Project Editor: Billy Fields
Copy Editor: Kevin Kent
Indexer: Johnna VanHoose Dinse
Interior Design and Layout: Katy Bodenmiller

DEDICATION

We dedicate this book to nurses across the globe who volunteer their time and talents to improve health and the quality of life for people worldwide.

ACKNOWLEDGEMENTS

Nurses around the world reach beyond their professional work to improve the lives of those in great need. Fortunately for us, many of those nurses have inspired our work and helped in the creation of this book. They have generously shared their wisdom with us, and we are most grateful.

Without mentors, we would not have become the nurses and volunteers we are today. We have worked with many nurses across the globe, and we thank them for their trust, collaboration, partnership, and friendship. First, we wish to thank those nurses who helped us as we began our own volunteer paths. Jeanne was inspired to reach beyond her work and her home by Jane Kallaus, MS, PNP, and Donna Schwartz-Barcott, PhD, RN, both of whom were inspirational teachers and mentors. The late Ruth Waldman, MS, RN—who worked with Intercultural Nursing, Inc.—Catherine Humphreys, MS, RN, and Jean Maher, MS, RN, helped shape Jeanne's beginning work with nursing students. Julia was inspired by nursing education leaders Sr. Madeleine Clemence Vaillot, OP, PhD, RN, who helped her learn that anything was possible to achieve, and Patricia Slater, MA, FRCN, College of Nursing, Australia, who was a change agent for nursing education.

We wish to thank those nurses around the world who partner with volunteer nurses and have helped all nurses improve their service at home and abroad. We personally wish to thank those nurses we have met in our local and global service, those we worked with around the world, and the students who helped Jeanne see the world through their eyes. We would love to name you all personally, but there are hundreds of you! Know that this book would not have been written without your generous contributions to our work.

In particular, we wish to thank Rhonda Martin, MPH, RN, and Mary Pat Couig, MPH, RN, FAAN, who helped us write Chapters 5, 7, and 8. Rhonda generously shared her expertise as a nurse in a travel medicine clinic, and Mary Pat shared her knowledge of disaster response from her expertise in the United States Public Health Service.

We sought to include the voices of nurses around the world, and we cannot thank our contributors enough for their willingness to share their words of wisdom with us. Some of these nurses are featured in the book; others offered help in a variety of ways that includes helping us make connections with other nurse volunteers, sending materials that we could learn from or use as reference materials in the book, and speaking with us on the telephone from points near and far. We thank them all for their expertise and continuing global service.

During the writing of this book, more than 20 of these nurses were actually serving as volunteers in their home countries and in Zambia, Uganda, Haiti, the Dominican Republic, and Nicaragua. We are grateful for the wisdom and contributions that the following nurses shared with us: Jean White, June Clark, Elizabeth Rosser, Anne Mason, Annabella Gloucester, Clare Lawrance, Marie Walters, Andrew Clarke, Suzanne Hardy, Joy Merrell, Pamela Llewellyn, Wim Breeman, Petra Frankhuizen, Hester Klopper, Lyn Middleton, Gerard M. Fealy, Damilie Mwogererwa, Speciosa Mbabali, Elizabeth

Ayebare, Scovia Mbalinda, Julia Samuelson, Lu Shek Eric Chan, Diane Martins, Alicia Curtin, Ruth McDermott-Levy, Elizabeth Keech, Amy Cory, Rita Ailinger, Gena Deck, Emma Mitchell, Mary Vrana, Stephanie Victoria, Amanda Nickerson, Jenna Domenici, Nicole DeMelo, Linda Baumann, Evelyn Gaudrault, Megan Smith, Myriam Jeannis, Ellen Milan, Michelle Belletete, Tamara McKinnon, Donna Nickitas, Karen Pehrson, and the members of the 2007-09 International Service Learning Task Force of the Honor Society of Nursing, Sigma Theta Tau International (STTI) and the STTI Region 15 Global Initiatives Committee for their wisdom and support to connect with nurses worldwide.

We could not have accomplished the work without the help of the editorial staff at STTI. Janet Boivin provided enthusiastic guidance and attention that was helpful at each phase of the work on this book. Carla Hall and the entire editorial staff offered insightful suggestions to the written word. We were indeed most fortunate to work with this talented team.

Jeanne's volunteer work would not have been possible without the support of her family. She is deeply grateful to her husband, Jim, and her children, Matt, John, and Annie, for their support for her volunteer work throughout her nursing career. Without Jim's loving support, Jeanne would not been able to complete this book.

Julia's career in nursing and her volunteer activities would not have been possible without the loving support of her late husband, Harold, and her children, Jeremy, Michael, Andrew, and Sheila, for which she will be forever grateful. Some of her assignments while in the U.S. Public Health Service were for extended periods of time, and her family always came together and supported each other during her long absences.

CONTRIBUTORS

IRELAND

Gerard M. Fealy, Associate Professor/Head of Research & Innovation Director, UCD Irish Centre for Nursing & Midwifery History, UCD School of Nursing, Midwifery & Health Systems, University College Dublin

NETHERLANDS

Wim Breeman, RN, CRNA, CFRN, EMT-P, M, ANP, Nurse Practitioner, Emergency Care

Petra Frankhuizen, RN, MANP, Ambulance Nurse

SOUTH AFRICA

Hester Klopper, PhD, MBA, RN, RM, Head of School of Nursing Science, North-West University

Lyn Middleton, Faculty of Health Sciences, Chair: Research Ethics and Higher Degrees Committee, University of KwaZulu-Natal

UNITED KINGDOM

Dame June Clark, DBE, RN, RHV, FRNC, FAAN, Professor Emerita, Swansea University, Wales

Andrew Clarke, RN, RHV, MPH, Health Advisor: Practice and Development, London and Nepal

Clare Lawrance, BSN, MN, Nurse Educator, VSO

Pamela Llewellyn, RGN, BSc, Community Health/District Nursing (UK)

Anne Mason, Lecturer, University of Stirling, Inverness, Scotland

Joy Merrell, Professor of Public Health Nursing, School of Human and Health Sciences, Swansea University, Singleton Park, Swansea, Wales

Elizabeth Rosser, RN, RM, DPhil, MN, DipRM, DipNEd, Dean at Bournemouth University

Marie Walters, BSN, MPH, Senior Lecturer, University of Wolverhampton

Jean White, Acting Chief Nurse Officer, Welch Assembly Governments

UGANDA

Elizabeth Ayebare, RN, PgD, Makarere University, Kampala

Speciosa Mbabali, RN, MSN, Chairperson of Nursing School, Makarere University, Kampala (retired)

Damalie Mwogererwa, URM, Mulago Hospital, Kampala

UNITED STATES OF AMERICA

Rita Ailinger, PhD, RN, Professor Emerita, George Mason University, Fairfax, VA

Linda Baumann, PhD, RN, FAAN, Professor, University of Wisconsin, Madison, WI

Michelle Belletete, BSN, former President of Intercultural Nursing, Inc., Jaffrey, NH

Amy Cory, PhD, RN, PNP, Assistant Professor, Valparaiso University, Valparaiso, IN

Mary Pat Couig, MPH, RN, FAAN, Rear Admiral, USPHS (retired), Intermittent Program Manager for the Office of Nursing Services, Veterans Health Administration

Alicia Curtin, PhD, GNP, Associate Professor, University of Rhode Island

Regena Deck, BS, RN, Emergency Department Nurse, Raymond, NH

Evelyn Gaudrault, MA, RN, Founder, Intercultural Nursing, Inc.

Myriam Jeannis, Senior Nursing Student, University of Massachusetts Dartmouth

Elizabeth Keech, PhD, RN, Assistant Professor, Villanova University

Rhonda Martin, MPH, RN, Critical Care and Travel Medicine Clinic Nurse, Boston, MA

Diane Martins, PhD, RN, Associate Professor, University of Rhode Island

Ruth McDermott-Levy, PhD, RN, Assistant Professor, Villanova University

Tamara McKinnon, MSN, RN, Lecturer in Nursing, San Jose State University

Ellen Milan, RNC, Neonatal Intensive Care Nurse, Florida

Emma Mitchell, PhD, RN, University of Virginia, Charlottesville, VA

Donna Nickitas, PhD, CNAA, BC, RN, Professor, Hunter College, New York, NY

Megan Smith, BSN, RN, Pediatric Nurse, Billerica, MA

Mary Vrana, BSN, RN, Medical Surgical Nurse, Providence, RI

Stephanie Victoria, BS, RN, Oncology Nurse, Boston, MA

WHO, Geneva, Switzerland

Julia Samuelson, HTM/HIV Dept/Prevention in the Health Sector, World Health Organization

Lu Shek Eric Chan, PhD, RN, Acting Chief Nursing Officer, WHO Headquarters

ABOUT THE AUTHORS

JEANNE M. LEFFERS, PHD, RN

Jeanne Leffers is currently professor of nursing at the University of Massachusetts Dartmouth in Dartmouth, Massachusetts, where she teaches in the undergraduate and graduate programs in nursing and serves the College of Nursing with her expertise in public health, environmental health, and global heath. Formerly she was the graduate program director. She has been actively involved with the Center for Teaching Excellence at the university by promoting faculty development for diversity initiatives, teaching and working to strengthen the academic programs in sustainable development with the Sustainability Program, and engaging university students in global learning with the International Student Programs. She has taught collaborative courses in the Sociology/Anthropology department and in the Sustainability Program.

A graduate of Simmons College School of Nursing, she completed her MS in nursing at the University of Rhode Island, and her MA and PhD in sociology at Brown University. During her professional nursing career, she worked with women and children and held positions as a public health nurse in Tennessee and Virginia prior to her 27 years in nursing education. She has taught at the University of Rhode Island and at University of Massachusetts Dartmouth.

Jeanne has published in the areas of public health nursing, environmental health, and global health. With funding from Health Care Without Harm, she has been instrumental in the development of the Knowledge Network, an online resource for nurses to learn essential knowledge for environmental health and to network with nurse colleagues to promote healthy environments. Additionally, she continues her work on partnerships and sustainability for global health nursing.

Jeanne is an active member of nursing organizations devoted to public health nursing, the nursing profession and nursing research. She has served on the executive board of the Association of Community Health Nursing Educators (ACHNE), as treasurer of Delta Upsilon-at-Large Chapter and as past president of Theta Kappa Chapter of Sigma Theta Tau International, and in other roles for the American Public

Health Nursing Association Public Health Nursing section, the Rhode Island State Nurses Association, and the Eastern Nursing Research Society. Currently, Jeanne is on the Steering Committee of the Alliance of Nurses for Healthy Environments (ANHE) and the Nursing Education Task Force of Health Volunteers Overseas, where she is the nurse coordinator for the nursing education program in Uganda. She serves on the Dean's Advisory Committee for Simmons College School for Health Sciences. Locally, she serves on the board of directors for the Greater New Bedford Community Health Center and the VNA of Southeastern Massachusetts.

Jeanne is the recipient of the University of Massachusetts Dartmouth Drum Major Award, the Simmons College Distinguished Alumna Award, the Genesis Award, and the Theta Kappa Chapter Leader Award.

JULIA R. PLOTNICK, MPH, RN, FAAN

Julia Plotnick earned a diploma from St. Anne's Hospital School of Nursing, a BSN from Catholic University, an MPH from the University of Pittsburgh, and a Pediatric Nurse Practitioner Certificate from Rutgers University. She served in the U.S. Public Health Service from 1959 to 1964 and again from 1979 to her retirement in 1996. As a community health and maternal/child specialist in that service, she held various national positions and accepted special international assignments to the World Health Organization. In 1992, the surgeon general of the Public Health Service selected Rear Admiral Plotnick as the chief nurse officer and assistant surgeon general. In her capacity as chief nurse, she was the principal advisor to the government on nursing affairs. She has served as an international consultant in numerous countries and represented the United States on the Global Advisory Group on Nursing to the director-general of the World Health Organization.

During her career, Julia was assigned to such disastrous situations as the famine in Sudan in 1988, the orphanage situation in Romania that came to light after the revolution of 1990, and the genocide in Rwanda in 1994. On these assignments, she used her past experiences, her intuition, and her initiative to bring positive results for each situation.

Upon retirement from the Public Health Service, Julia accepted the position of assistant to the director of the New Jersey Collaborating Center for Nursing at Rutgers University. In that role, she provided support and counsel for the executive director and also acted as an external liaison between the center and the nursing community. She also served as a part-time visiting professor at Rutgers College of Nursing. In 2001, she became a volunteer for Health Volunteers Overseas and initiated the first nursing volunteer activity for that organization in Uganda. She returned to Uganda several times, each time strengthening the program and encouraging other nurses to volunteer their time and expertise.

Julia serves on numerous boards in her retirement. She represented the U.S. Public Health Service on the executive board of the Military Officers Association of America. She was a founding member of the Commissioned Officers Foundation Board and served as the treasurer for 6 years. Julia is a consultant on African health affairs to the Foreign Service Institute, U.S. Department of State. She has served as a founding member of the Health Committee for the International Rescue Committee since 1997. She has served on the board of Health Volunteers Overseas since 2008 and currently serves as board chair.

In 2010, Julia was granted an honorary Doctor of Science degree from the University of Massachusetts Dartmouth. She was recognized for this high honor for her leadership, her nursing excellence and her commitment to public health and social justice.

She has received numerous awards and citations, including the Audrey Hepburn Humanitarian Award from Sigma Theta Tau International, the Outstanding Alumni Award from Catholic University of America, the Surgeon General's Medallion, and the Distinguished Service Medal, the highest honor of the U.S. Public Health Service.

REAR ADMIRAL MARY PAT COUIG, MPH, RN, FAAN

Mary Pat Couig completed her active duty career in the U.S. Public Health Service (PHS) as an assistant surgeon general and the chief professional officer for the nurse category. As a senior health care executive, she developed policy and provided leadership to both the Commissioned Corps and Civil Service nurses in the PHS. She worked closely with the Office of the Surgeon General and senior leadership in the Department of Health and Human Services, and was actively engaged in the development and implementation of national and global public health initiatives. Currently, she is an intermittent program manager for the Office of Nursing Services, Veterans Health Administration, and consults for federal agencies and contractors and professional organizations in public health preparedness, public health, and public health nursing.

During her PHS career, she was a member of the Federal Nursing Services Council, comprised of the nurse directors of the Air Force, Army, Navy, PHS, Veterans Health Administration and American Red Cross. From December 2000 until October 2005, her collaborative efforts with the Federal Nursing Services Council and local, state, national, and international colleagues focused on strengthening nursing's role and preparation for public health preparedness. The secretary of health and human services appointed her as the field commander for Emergency Support Function #8, Public Health and Medical, during Hurricane Rita in 2005.

Couig received her BSN from Fitchburg State College in Fitchburg, Massachusetts, and her Master's in Public Health from Johns Hopkins School of Hygiene and Public Health, Baltimore, Maryland. She is enrolled in the doctoral nursing program at the Uniformed Services University of the Health Sciences in Bethesda, Maryland.

RHONDA MARTIN, MPH, RN

Rhonda Martin's nursing career has spanned 30 years in clinical, managerial, and research roles. Currently, she is a critical care nurse and travel medicine clinic nurse in the Boston area. Through her years in nursing, her love of remote adventure travel and exploring cultural diversity, alongside a career as an intensive care, emergency room, and travel medicine nurse, have come together in her global nursing missions.

Her first global nursing mission was in Tanzania as a nursing student, where she resided in a leprosarium and visited remote villages with a public health nurse. The seed was planted and subsequently, Rhonda has worked in the Dominican Republic with Intercultural Nursing and in Rwanda with Team Heart Rwanda. Currently, she has her own program for teaching and mentoring hospital nurses in Katmandu, Nepal. In addition, Rhonda has worked in disaster response, most recently when deployed to Mississippi after Hurricane Katrina in 2005.

She received her BSN from Pacific Lutheran University, an MPH in the global health track from the University of Texas, and a post-graduate diploma in travel medicine from the University of Glasgow, Scotland.

TABLE OF CONTENTS

PROLOGUE. OR, WHAT BROUGHT US TO THIS WORK.

JEANNE'S STORY

Throughout my childhood, high school, and college years, I dreamed of becoming a nurse who served those most disadvantaged. This desire led me to volunteer during my high school and college years not only in hospitals, but also in nursing homes, inner city community centers, and evolving community health centers, and also as a tutor. As a senior nursing student, I was privileged to have the opportunity to spend 1 month of my community health practicum living and working with migrant farm workers in upstate New York. It was here that my youthful dreams grew into a passion for the underserved.

I had to put my dream of serving internationally on hold for the next few decades because of professional and family demands. Professionally, I worked in a variety of settings, primarily as a public health nurse and for the past 27 years, as college of nursing faculty. During this time, I continued my community service in a variety of settings. The one that best positioned me for global nursing was 7 years of service to the Genesis Center, a Providence, Rhode Island, a family multi-service center for immigrants and refugees to learn English and job training skills. As a volunteer nurse, I assisted center applicants with common health problems, created health education programs, and guided them in their efforts to seek health care in their new environment. They represented more than 20 different countries from Latin America, Asia, Africa, and Eastern Europe. My work as a volunteer nurse helped me learn about their cultural practices, health beliefs, and needs as new immigrants to the United States.

When the timing was right for me to travel internationally, I began a journey of more than 15 years to become a more effective global volunteer. In my first two assignments, I spent about 10 days each in Guatemala and the Dominican Republic, learning how to be a nurse volunteer in a country where the language and culture differed from my own. Fortunately, my years of work with many Guatemalans and Dominicans in Providence helped me to be more sensitive to their particular cultural needs. Additionally, I studied development and comparative health systems during my graduate studies in sociology, building my knowledge of the impact of history, culture, politics, and economics upon health.

In my faculty role, I find that students continually request international nursing experience, but they find it challenging to meet this goal within the structured undergraduate curriculum. Beginning in 1999, using a Feinstein Service Learning grant with another University of Rhode Island faculty colleague, the late Ruth Waldman, MS, RN, and I worked to develop a 2-week immersion experience for students in collaboration with Intercultural Nursing, Inc. Students traveled to the Dominican Republic as part of a team of nurses, other health professionals, and interpreters to improve health access and care in a remote region of the country. Since that time, I have traveled with more than 60 nursing students to the Dominican Republic, Haiti, and Honduras. During a sabbatical in 2008, I sought a long-term assignment that focused upon capacity building for those with whom I would work. Finding a match with Health Volunteers Overseas, I traveled to Uganda to collaborate with nurses at Mulago Hospital and with the nursing faculty and students at Makerere University.

Throughout these years, I became convinced that the most effective nurse volunteer works in a program that matches nurse expertise and program needs, takes the time to learn about what the host partners want from volunteers, partners with local health care providers, and works collaboratively to empower others to meet their own needs. With deep respect for the people I have had the privilege to learn from and care for at home and in countries far from home, I encourage you, as a potential nurse volunteer, to use the information we offer in this book to create the best volunteer experience for you and to become the best volunteer you can be.

JULIA'S STORY

As long as I can remember, I wanted to be a nurse. I was the youngest of six children. My father died when I was 11 and my mother, a teacher by profession, worked long and hard to educate all of us. Because of college costs for my older siblings, my mother suggested that I do the diploma nursing program at the local hospital and then continue on for my bachelor in nursing immediately after graduation, when she would be better able to assist me.

My mother was the ultimate community volunteer. In the early 1900s, she organized classes for new immigrants, teaching English and life skills. She established women's clubs and women's guilds that offered support for new mothers and classes in cooking, child care, and health, as well as other projects. She encouraged all of her children to give of themselves and share with others. Each in our own way has followed her example.

As a new nurse, my first solo volunteer activity was to start a Girl Scout troop for hospitalized, emotionally disturbed girls ages 9-12. It was a moderately successful project, but a real challenge. It made me understand how much I still had to learn! My next foray into volunteering was in Turkey. My husband was on a 1-year sabbatical in Ankara, Turkey. Armed with a new Master's in Public Health, I met with the Ministry of Health and offered to start health centers in three small villages near Ankara. Two American nurses joined me and during that year, we successfully established the centers, traveling to them every week with a Turkish doctor and an interpreter.

Educational and family commitments filled a few ensuing years. When the pediatric nurse practitioner program became available in the late 1960s, I knew this was an ideal path for me. With this new certificate, one community health worker and I, with some federal funding, opened a free neighborhood pediatric clinic that was open several evenings a week. It proved to be so successful that the County Health Department took it over as a permanent part of their service.

When I was able to return to full-time employment, I rejoined the United States Public Health Service. I was assigned to a medically underserved, health-manpower shortage area as the pediatric nurse practitioner and public health nurse. This was a most rewarding assignment for me. The opportunities for volunteering for me and for my children were tremendous.

During my career in the Public Health Service, I was given many short-term assignments throughout the world, mainly during catastrophic situations where mothers and children were unduly affected. These included the famine in Sudan, the Romanian orphanage situation, the Nicaraguan refugee migration on the Texas-Mexican border, the hurricanes that affected the United States coastal states, the aftermath of the Rwandan genocide, and many others. On each and every assignment, I learned so much more than I was able to offer. Each assignment built on the previous one. So many times on assignment, the resiliency of the human spirit of the mothers and children who were affected encouraged me to do my very best to alleviate their suffering.

In retirement, I continue to volunteer my time by serving on several boards of nongovernmental organizations, such as International Rescue Committee, Women's Commission for Refugee Women and Children, Health Volunteers Overseas, and others. This provides me with a great opportunity to speak of the value of nurse volunteers and to encourage my nursing colleagues to offer their knowledge and expertise in a most rewarding way.

INTRODUCTION
WHY THIS BOOK IS IMPORTANT

Our purpose in writing this book is to offer essential information for nurses who volunteer globally. By this, we mean that nurses may volunteer within the boundaries of their own home country or travel to countries beyond their borders. While some (Collins, DeZerenga, & Heckscher, 2002) refer to global volunteering as service that occurs beyond the boundaries of one's own home country, we recognize that increasing diversity of populations worldwide, growing health disparities, and human needs in one's own home country encourage nurses to seek to volunteer at home. What we offer in this book will be helpful to nurses making decisions about volunteering in any setting. In addition, nurse volunteers often travel to another location in their own country or abroad for little or no pay, to provide nursing expertise to those in need (Collins, DeZerenga, & Heckscher, 2002). Therefore, we consider that nurses who assume roles for little or no pay or respond to the need to serve beyond their defined employment will find this book helpful to their work.

In each setting, the professional nurse is stepping beyond his or her regular professional role to take on an assignment to improve health for those in other settings. This can be as near to home as working with people who are homeless in one's own community or traveling thousands of miles to help those who struggle with issues of poverty, malnutrition, and limited access to health care. Some of our readers may have many years of experience with volunteer service, some may have been contemplating making a volunteer commitment for the first time, and some may be responding to human need in times of disaster. Nurses serve people and communities in many ways, but in our profession we are often the catalysts that inspire others as well. By becoming effective volunteers, nurses make an impact upon health far beyond the immediate services rendered.

WHO SHOULD READ THIS BOOK?

Increasingly, nurses travel to locations in response to disasters and to serve with international service organizations. We specifically speak to nurses who respond to disasters near and far, nurses who undertake short-term volunteer assignments in their home country, nurses who wish to travel overseas to volunteer, and nurses who work with service-learning programs with student participants. We do not limit our focus to one type of nurse but consider the breadth of expertise nurses possess as skilled clinicians, educators, researchers, consultants, administrators, and policymakers. In addition, we consider the special topics that might relate to nursing students, newly licensed nurses, nurses who practice in highly specialized clinical areas, and nurses who are about to or have retired from active nursing practice.

HOW WE CAME TO DO THIS WORK

We bring many years of experience as nursing volunteers in our communities and as nurses who have worked in a variety of countries beyond our home in the United States. We offer the reader more information about our personal experiences and stories throughout the book. What is important to us as authors is that our work has brought us wonderful opportunities to engage with nurses around the world who have made substantial contributions to this book. Their stories and expertise enrich the book. We could not have done this work without the collective wisdom of nurses worldwide.

WHAT WE DO IN THE BOOK

Our goal in this book is to offer a combination of practical information and larger ethical concerns to frame nurse volunteering. You will find practical information to aid in your decision-making about whether to volunteer, how to prepare to be an effective volunteer, and advice about logistical issues prior to and during the assignment. Beyond this essential knowledge that helps you learn how to do this work, we discuss issues important for nurses to consider as global citizens of the world. By this we mean that we have learned, from our 40 collective years in global health nursing, that our service extends beyond the weeks or months we may actually serve. Our service can promote partnership and sustainability (Leffers & Mitchell, 2011), as well as empower nurses globally to improve health. We speak to the importance of culturally sensitive, ethical, and legal nursing practice that upholds the highest practice standards for all people worldwide. Meeting these standards also includes consideration of the use of appropriate technology, medications, medical waste, and respect for the local environment.

Part 1: History and Perspectives of Nurse Volunteering

Global health nursing is not a recent phenomenon; it dates back to Florence Nightingale and the beginning of the profession. As travel became easier, technology provided the means to connect people worldwide, and the number of volunteer opportunities increased, greater numbers of nurses elected to volunteer in distant settings. In this section, we situate the current opportunities for nurses within the larger history of global nursing service.

Part 2: Making the Decision to Volunteer

We offer the reader information that will help the potential or seasoned volunteer make important decisions about how to use specific talents and nursing expertise. In addition we explain how to locate a program that is the best fit for their particular talents. Through these chapters, we address volunteer situations where the nurse serves as an educator to partners in the host setting, as a clinician providing direct care to people living in the host setting, or as a consultant to nurses or other health professionals in a host setting. This includes Chapter 2, "Thinking Seriously About Volunteering," which provides tools for self-assessment to help the reader identify nursing expertise, skills, goals, and needs in a volunteer assignment. Next, in Chapter 3, "Finding a Volunteer Program," we provide information that will guide the reader to assess potential volunteer opportunities. We identify where most volunteers can learn about opportunities, the mission and goals of organizations, nursing roles, and special factors such as travel, cost, and living arrangements. Finally, in Chapter 4, "Matching Your Self-Assessment and Program Needs: Finding the Best Fit," we help you determine the best match for you in planning your volunteer opportunity.

Part 3: Special Volunteer Opportunities

In Chapter 5, "Nursing Response to Disasters," and Chapter 6, "Experiential Learning for Faculty and Student Nurses," we address particular subsets of nurses who serve in these roles. We consulted with Mary Patricia Couig, MPH, RN, FAAN, RADM, USPHS (Ret.), an expert in nurse participation in disaster response, to offer essential information in Chapter 5 for nurses who respond to both local and global disasters. Since the preparation time for travel to a disaster setting is short and information about the role of the nurse, living conditions, and needs of those affected by the disaster is limited, we offer advice about disaster nursing that supplements what is offered in Chapters 2, 3 and 4.

In addition, there is a growing emphasis upon global health and service learning for nursing education (Sigma Theta Tau International Service Learning Task Force, 2009). Increasingly, schools and colleges of nursing respond to their university mission and goals that emphasize global citizenry and international educational programs. Faculty members with experience in global service seek to create opportunities for their students to grow professionally and personally from this rewarding work. In addition, students themselves also seek opportunities for global service learning and encourage faculty and administration at their schools to provide them. Drawing from more than 10 years of experience with international service learning, and using examples shared by nursing faculty around the United States, Jeanne offers important knowledge for those planning student global nursing experiences.

Part 4: Planning for and Completing the Volunteer Assignment

Here we deal with practical information about preparation for the trip, the actual volunteer experience, and coming home. We address important personal issues of emotional and physical well-being, how to become an effective volunteer, important partnership issues for the host country or location, and what to expect when you return home. Rhonda Martin, MPH, RN, shared her expertise as a nurse in a travel medicine clinic to provide extensive information on health and safety in volunteer settings. Integrated with our practical guidance are the important issues that promote ethical and responsible service.

"CHANGING LIVES" FEATURE

Throughout the book, we include features from nursing colleagues around the world who share their stories and knowledge to help you learn from their experience. Though we speak from our perspective as American nurses, we aim to project a global voice from nurses worldwide. To hear perspectives of nurses still in the early years of volunteer service as well as global health experts, we include nurses who only began their volunteer journey during the past 12 months, in addition to those who have decades of service. These features will provide you with richer insights into global volunteering.

TOOLS AND RESOURCES

Throughout the book, we offer tools to help you select the best volunteer opportunity for yourself. These include a set of self-assessment questions, a checklist for identification of important factors in a volunteer organization, and a guide to help you determine the fit between your self-assessment and the volunteer program you have selected. We provide a number of logistical tips in the form of a packing list, tips for personal health and safety, strategies that address cultural differences, and appendices for resources relevant to international travel, nurse volunteering, service learning, and cultural factors that impact health.

HOW TO USE THIS BOOK EFFECTIVELY

While we arranged the material in sequential order from the self-assessment phase to your return home from the volunteer assignment, the reader can elect to begin reading anywhere. For example, if you have already committed to an organization and specified role, you may decide to begin with the logistical and practical information about preparation and the actual volunteer experience in Chapters 7 and 8. We do urge the reader to then return to the early chapters to learn more about how to become the most effective volunteer one can be. Additionally, the special features we use to share the wisdom of our nursing colleagues are likely to provide information that extends the breadth and depth of what we have provided.

We also suggest that you read the book with a notebook nearby to record important information, to pose questions you have so you can return to locate answers, and to respond to the questions that we pose. Our goal is to provide you with the most comprehensive information to help you determine if volunteering is for you and to prepare for a volunteer assignment. Speaking not only for ourselves but for the thousands of nurses who volunteer, we know that this volunteer work brings rewards and memories that last a lifetime.

REFERENCES

Collins, J., DeZerega, S., & Heckscher, Z. (2002). *How to live your dream of volunteering overseas.* New York: Penguin.

Leffers, J., & Mitchell, E. (2011). Conceptual model for partnership and sustainability in global health. *Public Health Nursing, 28*(1), 98-102.

Sigma Theta Tau International Service Learning Task Force. (2009). *Service learning: Pedagogy of civic engagement for nursing.* Unpublished manuscript.

CHAPTER 1

HISTORY AND PERSPECTIVES OF NURSE VOLUNTEERING

Nurse volunteering is as old as the nursing profession. Florence Nightingale, held to be the founder of nursing, led her team of 38 nurses into Scutari, Turkey, during the Crimean War of 1854 (Dossey, 2010; Gill, 2004). The nurse volunteer in times of war continues to the current day. Most countries do not issue conscription for nurses, and nurses volunteer to join the military and serve where needed. In the United States, beginning with the Civil War of 1861–1865, Dorothea Dix, a non-nurse, advocated for nurses to serve the wounded. She was assigned the duty of building a nurse team for this service. Thousands of nurses responded, and she selected 2,000 nurses to serve during that war. As the war continued, the numbers of nurses serving increased as well ("Northern volunteer nurses," 2011).

Clara Barton, not a trained nurse but considered a nurse leader, founded the American Red Cross in 1882 in affiliation with the International Red Cross in Europe. This organization engaged nurses as volunteers during the yellow fever outbreak in Florida in 1888; the Johnstown, Pennsylvania, flood of 1889 that killed more than 2,000 people and left 25,000 homeless; and the Spanish-American War, where more than 700 nurses served (Allgeyer, 2011).

By 1909, nurse Jane Delano was appointed as director of the American Red Cross and created a Red Cross nurses' reserve to prepare nurses to serve in military roles in times of war. By 1918, this reserve of nurses was crucial to serving those affected by the Spanish Flu epidemic. More than 15,000 nurses volunteered at that time with the American Red Cross (Allgeyer, 2011). After World War I, many countries launched military nursing organizations, such as the Army Nurse Corps in the United States. By World War II, more than 60,000 volunteer army nurses served ("What role," 2011).

Throughout the history of the International Red Cross, nurses volunteered to serve in disasters and continue to do so to this day. In Chapter 5 we address particular issues for nurse volunteers who serve in times of disaster. Retired or inactive nurses can be potential volunteers during such a time of need (Fothergill, Palumbo, Rambur, Reinier, & McIntosh, 2005).

NURSES AS VOLUNTEERS

Since the early days of the nursing profession, nurses have served as volunteers at home and abroad. Currently, the growth of opportunities for nurse volunteers provides us with ways to broaden our professional skills while serving others. Further, at times, a role that nurses assume as volunteers is so valuable to an organization that the organization creates a permanent and reimbursed position. The unique abilities of nurses, as well as our range of professional skills, position us for volunteering in many venues.

WHY ARE NURSES SO SUITED TO VOLUNTEER ROLES?

The characteristics that are often ascribed to nurses are consistent with the qualities that make good volunteers. Nurses are described as compassionate, empathetic, and respectful of those they care for. Nurses need to have energy and endurance, effective interpersonal and communication skills, and problem-solving skills, and they need to pay close attention to detail. Additionally, nurses must have emotional maturity, flexibility, and adaptability to deal with unexpected situations. As scientists, nurses bring knowledge to assist in many venues where volunteers are needed. Further, the art of nursing allows nurses to creatively care for people holistically by meeting them at their points of need.

Collins, DeZerega, and Hecksher (2002) list five character traits of highly effective volunteers:

- They have *flexibility* to do what is necessary rather than simply enacting their own plans or grandiose dreams.

- *Patience* is required not only to adjust to cultural differences in timeliness for meetings with local partners or to deal with the lack of equipment necessary for efficient work, but also in terms of the need to proceed slowly to collaborate and move a project forward.

- *Openness* is essential. This begins with tolerance and respect and can lead you to try new ways of social interactions and to accept alternative healing modalities.

- Volunteers must be *dependable*. Be present when you promise to be, show up on time, and follow through on your assigned tasks. Your host partners are also investing time for the work and need volunteers to be committed and dependable.

- Effective volunteers must have *humility*. Volunteers must recognize that, though they might be experts at home, in the host setting they are novices. Later in this chapter we will offer an example of nurse volunteer Diane Martins to illustrate this type of service. She would explain that even though she is a highly educated and skilled nurse, she would not know how to survive one cold night on the street.

As nurses we build relationships with those we care for and learn from their spirit and our engagement in their lives. As a first-year student at Simmons College in Boston, Jeanne took on the responsibility of chairing the freshman class project. The project provided an opportunity for the freshmen to see firsthand what life was like in the Bromley Heath housing project, a place only a short mile away physically but worlds apart from the rich academic, scientific, and cultural institutions of the campus. The student volunteers agreed that they learned a great deal about the strengths and resilience of others from their relationship with residents there, but they also learned a great deal about themselves. It is this, we believe, that is at the core of why nurses volunteer: because we know that through our service to others, we learn about ourselves and enjoy the rewards of working with other people in need.

What about when nurses step into another environment one that might be as close physically as the housing project Jeanne worked with, but one that is far distant from the nurse's experience? The following sidebar, the experience of Diane Martins, PhD, RN, serves as an example of a nurse who has volunteered for more than 30 years in her local community.

CHANGING LIVES

Diane Martins is an example of a nurse who has been a volunteer in her local community for more than 30 years, despite her full-time employment in other practice settings. As a young nurse at St. Vincent's Hospital in New York City, she saw many patients come into the intensive care unit where she worked who did not have homes to return to upon discharge. Often their admission occurred because of hypothermia or sequelae of living on the streets. She elected to learn more about these patients, those referred to as "bag ladies" and "runaway kids," by volunteering at local soup kitchens.

Diane moved from NYC to Rhode Island about 30 years ago and continued to serve those living without homes in various ways. For more than 20 years, she was a regular volunteer on the mobile van that served the homeless population throughout the metropolitan Providence area. As the programs with Travelers Aid grew, she served as one of more than 100 doctors and nurses working with the van, in the inner city clinic and service center, or at the Welcome Arnold Shelter. She served on the board for the Rhode Island Coalition for the Homeless to work toward better programs to improve health and safety. During this time her full-time position was as a community health nursing faculty member at the University of Rhode Island. She negotiated placements for nursing students in the various programs that served those living on the streets and without homes. Hundreds of nursing students learned about health care issues for the homeless and many became advocates, volunteers, or care providers for the homeless themselves.

VOLUNTEERING LOCALLY

Arthur Blaustein, author of *Make a Difference: America's Guide to Volunteering and Community Service* (2003), notes that community service and citizen participation have been fundamental to American culture since the founding of the country in 1776. In the book, Blaustein provides a compilation of volunteer opportunities across the spectrum of human needs. Explaining that community service is a two-way street of giving and receiving, he notes that former volunteers have used words such as human connection, learning, spiritual growth, enjoyable, and adventure to describe their experiences.

NURSE VOLUNTEERING EXAMPLES

Nurses continue to volunteer in times of disaster and in long-term assignments in their local communities. Some authors suggest that this is an important role for inactive nurses as well (Fothergill, Palumbo, Rambur, Reinier, & McIntosh, 2005).

Nurses reach out in many ways to volunteer—serving in immunization clinics, performing health screenings, and working at local schools. While these nurses assigned to specific volunteer roles may be less likely to need the guidance provided throughout this book, we believe that all nurse volunteers can benefit from reading the sections on ethical and responsible service.

What was formerly called parish nursing and is now more commonly referred to as faith community nursing frequently engages thousands of nurses as volunteers in their own faith setting. The roots of this movement in the United States began in Europe with the Deaconess nurses who served in the community, bringing nursing and spiritual care to those they served (Kreutzer, 2010). Begun in the 1980s in the United States in a new form, the movement has grown to include thousands of nurses serving in all faith communities. Nurses address health, wellness, wholeness, and healing in their own congregations through such interventions as health promotion programs, health advocacy, health care access, and navigation assistance, and through supportive relationships with members of their faith community. They achieve many of these goals through activities such as health fairs, blood pressure screenings, and the offering of referral services (Otterness, Gehrke & Sener, 2007). Since its inception, a number of programs to educate faith community nurses have been developed, and the American Nurses Association (ANA) and Health Ministries Association have developed the *Faith Community Nursing: Scope and Standards of Practice* (2005). This type of community nursing practice would not have grown to become the essential services seen today without the participation of many nurse volunteers (Brudenell, 2003; Lundy & Janes, 2009; Maurer & Smith, 2009).

NURSING IN A GLOBAL WORLD

Nurses also contribute to global health efforts by volunteering in international humanitarian settings. Frequently you will hear the terms *mission* or *health brigade* to describe global volunteer efforts. The term mission does not denote health care efforts solely under the auspices of religious groups but is a term often used to explain the short-term trips that health professionals embark upon to meet the needs of people worldwide. Nurses from the United States often serve with the SS *Hope* and in the Peace Corps. As travel and international opportunities increase, many nurses worldwide travel to other countries with organizations whose missions are to provide medical and nursing care to those in need (Crigger & Holcomb, 2007; Crump & Sugarman, 2010; Levi, 2009). We offer resources in Appendix A to help you learn more about global issues.

FAMOUS MODERN-ERA NURSE VOLUNTEERS

It's not just Florence Nightingale who is known worldwide for volunteer nurse service. Three modern-era volunteer nurses, all of whom traveled great distances and made an impact on international health, are detailed below.

Former U.S. President Jimmy Carter's mother was a nurse. His 2008 biography of her records not only her lifelong achievements but also her service in the Peace Corps in 1966 at age 68 (Carter, 2008). She believed in giving back and that you were never too old for volunteer work. Today, the Lillian Carter Center for International Nursing at Emory University serves a central position in the international health and midwifery work of the nursing program.

Claire Bertschinger, a nurse who currently runs the Diploma in Tropical Nursing certificate program at the

London School of Hygiene and Tropical Medicine became known for her work in Ethiopia during the famine in the mid-1980s. When musician Bob Geldof met her in Ethiopia, he was so moved by the humanitarian needs and by her work that he went on to create Live Aid, a worldwide concert to support the famine, and raised almost $300,000. Claire's book *Moving Mountains* (2005) follows her career of service to the International Red Cross from her early service up through her service in Uganda, Kenya, Afghanistan, and West Africa. When asked how such a gentle woman could make a difference in situations as difficult as the ones she encountered, she responded, "There's nothing sweeter, gentler, or softer than water ... but water had the ability to move mountains (Bertschinger & Blake, 2005, p. 15). Her words remind all nurses that efforts great or small can help to make big improvements.

Most recently, the public has read about nurse Greg Mortenson, the author of *Three Cups of Tea* and *Stones into Schools*, who began the Central Asia Institute (CAI) in response to the desired goal of the local people of Korphe, Pakistan, who ministered to him when he was lost and injured on a mountain climb up K2. His newfound friend, Haji Ali, asked for a school but first needed a bridge in order to get supplies to the region. Since his decision to help in 1993, Mortenson has led the institute in establishing or supporting more than 170 schools in Pakistan and Afghanistan, reaching more than 68,000 students. In addition, the CAI focuses its work on education, health issues, the environment, and cultural preservation. Examples of the work include training and support for teachers, building libraries, promoting women's educational and vocational training, and establishing scholarships, water projects, sanitation projects, and rural health care camps (Central Asia Institute, 2011; Mortenson, 2009; Mortenson & Relin, 2006). (Editor's Note: As this book was going to press in April 2011, reports surfaced that Greg Mortenson may have misreported events in his books regarding his travels and work in Afghanistan. In absence of definitive answers, readers may note that his work with the Central Asia Institute continues and has been influential in the region.)

Though nurses who embark on missions to help improve the health and welfare of those in distant countries are not likely to demonstrate the impact of these nurses, the education and knowledge they possess provide them with the important skills needed to make a difference. Lillian Carter, Claire Bertschinger, and Greg Mortenson all took that first small but courageous step before building their legacies.

GLOBALIZATION AND HEALTH

Nurse volunteering is affected by globalization. The term *globalization* refers to the social, political, economic, technological, and intellectual connections around the world (Wilson, 2011). We witness this regularly with the global market for production and trade, effects of the global economy, ability to communicate in real time across the globe through the Internet and other telecommunications, and the ease of travel not only for humans, but for goods and diseases. The rapid global changes brought on by globalization have a profound impact upon health. Though fears of a global pandemic of SARS or H1N1 influenza demonstrate the impact of globalization on health, other entities such as trade agreements, telecommunications, energy consumption, and food supplies all contribute to health or illness. International trade agreements such as the North American Free Trade Agreement (NAFTA) and the General Agreement on Trade in Services (GATS), among others, not only can improve the ability of governments to monitor and protect health, but also have such negative consequences as a government's ability to regulate food products, to regulate the environment, and to provide access to clean water and affordable medications (Shaffer, Waitzkin, Brenner, & Jasso-Aguilar, 2005).

Consequently, globalization affects the health of people worldwide directly and indirectly. Failing economies in poor countries increase nurse migration from those countries where their services are in great need to richer countries where there are better economic opportunities (Kingma, 2008; Rosenkoetter & Nardi, 2007). For example, the growing pandemic of HIV/AIDS is exacerbated by the ease with which microbes can spread globally. However, the impact of the economic recession occurring during the last years of the 2000–2010 decade has increased homelessness and hunger globally, has reduced the ability of families to pay school fees in countries where education is not guaranteed, and has negatively affected job opportunities for not only immigrants and the least educated but also across all sectors. As a result, nurse volunteers find increasing numbers of people in need at home and abroad.

GLOBAL HEALTH

Nurses who volunteer in all settings must be knowledgeable about the common health problems of the population they serve. Diane Martins, mentioned earlier in the chapter, works with a homeless population and must be skilled in dealing with people who suffer from exposure to the cold, from untreated chronic illnesses such as diabetes and hypertension, with mental health conditions, and with substance abuse problems. Nurses who elect to volunteer in poor tropical countries must learn about diseases such as malaria, dengue, schistosomiasis, skin conditions, and other tropical diseases.

Most often an organization where a nurse volunteers has completed an assessment of the population strengths and needs, but if one is not available, a nurse should complete a community assessment to work collaboratively with the population served. Nurses learn community assessment approaches in their baccalaureate education but we suggest that you consult Anderson and McFarlane (2011), Maurer and Smith (2009), and Stanhope and Lancaster (2008) to learn more about conducting a community assessment.

For nurses who serve abroad, the United Nations Millennium Declaration (2000) developed target goals for 2015 that address global health and well-being. These eight goals, called the Millennium Development Goals (MDGs), serve as universal goals for all countries to meet the needs of the poorest people in the world (see Box 1.1). Though obviously three of these goals are health targets, achievement of all eight of the goals will positively impact health (Millennium Development Goals, 2011).

BOX 1.1

MILLENNIUM DEVELOPMENT GOALS

Goal #1	End Hunger and Poverty
Goal #2	Achieve Universal Primary Education
Goal #3	Achieve Gender Equity and Empower Women
Goal #4	Reduce Child Mortality
Goal #5	Improve Maternal Health
Goal #6	Combat HIV/AIDS, Malaria, and Other Diseases
Goal #7	Ensure Environmental Sustainability
Goal #8	Develop a Global Partnership for Development

Nurse volunteers should all be aware of the target points for the MDGs. Additionally, they need to understand the leading global health problems. Though infectious diseases such as malaria, tuberculosis, HIV/AIDS, emerging infections, and drug-resistant variants of disease still ravage the poorer populations in the developing world, nurse volunteers need to note that chronic illnesses such as heart disease, diabetes, and cancer are increasing causes of mortality and morbidity worldwide. Additionally, in much of the developing world, road-traffic accidents are a growing problem that not only increases the mortality rate but also leaves victims with lifelong disabilities that are often difficult to treat in poorer parts of the world. Information specific to the country where the nurse volunteer will serve is available from the World Health Organization (WHO) website (http://www.who.int/research/en/).

ENVIRONMENT AND SUSTAINABILITY

First noted as essential to optimal health by Florence Nightingale, a healthy environment is necessary for health. Food-borne and water-borne illnesses have a significant impact worldwide but most profoundly in the poorest, least developed countries where nurse volunteers are likely to serve. Access to clean water, safe and healthy food, and basic sanitation to assure hygiene and lack of contamination are essential to health improvement and to meeting the MDGs. Films such as *Water First*, available from Bullfrog Films, link all of the MDGs with the need for clean water (http://www.waterfirstfilm.org/data/content/view/23/46/).

Yet the increasing environmental health issues globally are not always a top priority for global health missions. We have observed the increasing use of plastic for bags, water bottles, and packaging materials in poorer parts of the world. Though the benefits of clean bottled water are important in preventing biologic pathogens, most countries in the developing world burn their refuse, thus increasing the dispersion of carcinogens into the air, water, and soil. Additionally, motor vehicle congestion and minimal vehicular exhaust regulations contribute to poor air quality that negatively affects cardiac and respiratory health. Further, many countries lack regulations to protect the health of workers and the environment. As globalization demands increase manufacturing in poorer countries, more and more workers are exposed to potential toxins in the workplace, and improper disposal of hazardous waste can affect the health of communities. The organization Health Care Without Harm (www.noharm.org), developed in 1996 by nurses and other concerned professionals, works globally to address the rise of environmental threats to health and the environment.

Climate change adversely affects the most vulnerable, as demonstrated by increased drought and floods, the increase in infectious agents, and heat waves. The elderly, children, and those with altered immune systems are most at risk. Though nurse volunteers are unlikely to make significant changes to the environment in the volunteer setting, nurses can and should ensure that volunteer programs do not adversely affect the environment in the host setting. For example, many missions involve dispensing medications in small plastic bags and distributing donations in plastic bags. Reusable bags need to be part of every volunteer program so that the person receiving the bag of donations will have a reusable bag and thus reduce waste in the host country. Second, nurse volunteers need to consider the hazardous effects of pharmaceutical waste on the host country environment. Careful plans for medication use and disposal demonstrate respect for the local environment.

Finally, nurse volunteers who work collaboratively with nurse partners globally should educate themselves and their colleagues about the hazardous health effects present in the environment and about the steps they can take to ensure environmental sustainability. Nurse volunteers can use and recommend an accessible resource for nurses worldwide to learn about the latest information on environmental health nursing (www.envirn.org). This resource provides educational, advocacy, practice, and research resources for environmental health nursing and can be a valuable, accessible resource for global nurse partners.

ETHICAL AND RESPONSIBLE SERVICE

Julia and Jeanne have learned from years of volunteer service and the collective wisdom of our nurse colleagues that making a difference depends upon providing ethical and responsible service. Thankfully, we have yet to meet a nurse volunteer who did not have the best intentions. We want to encourage our readers to become volunteers, but we also want our readers to be aware of the ethical and cultural implications of volunteer nurse service. We have seen situations where the ethical principle of nonmaleficence, or "First do no harm," can be called into question. Critiques of health care missions argue that sometimes the efforts are likely to foster dependence (Levi, 2009), fail to address the long-term social and political causes of health inequalities (Crigger, 2008), and could be more likely to meet the needs of the volunteer than those being served (Crump & Sugarman, 2008). Crigger and Holcomb (2007) speak about ethical situations faced by nurses who volunteer in other countries that arise from working in a setting where cultural norms differ and from ethical dilemmas for nursing that arise in a different culture. Adequately trained volunteers who might lack cultural sensitivity and who fail to work with the local partners might indeed bring harm rather than help to those they are trying to serve. Throughout the book, we offer strategies to help you make the best decision for your volunteer assignment to use your expertise in the best program for you.

Examples of doing harm can be the use of medications not generally available in the host country and not used properly for any particular patients. Use of antibiotics can be helpful but also poses risks for antibiotic allergy and anaphylaxis as well as antibiotic resistance. Language translation may be a problem in ensuring proper administration of medications. For example, the English word *once* is also a Spanish word, *once*, meaning 11, which could account for an overdose of medication. When families live in small homes where there are children, safe storage of medications is a concern. Children can be at risk of an overdose of medication, particularly because many medications resemble candy. Finally, nurses are becoming more aware of the adverse health effects of improper disposal of medications (ANHE, 2010). Crigger and Holcomb (2007) recommend that individuals be educated on nonpharmacologic management first and that treatment with medications for chronic conditions be limited and require careful follow-up. They also suggest nurses administer only those medications available in the host country, use only medications that are available on the essential drug list published by the WHO, and administer only medications that are appropriate to clinical needs, in responsible doses to meet the patient's individual requirement, for the appropriate time, and at the lowest cost to them.

Crigger and Holcomb (2007) recommmend four strategies for more inclusive health care while volunteering in other countries:

- *Revealing ignorance* refers to the fact that no one can be culturally competent in a culture other than one's own, and by using the approach that recognizes what they do not know, nurses are likely to learn and better understand their partners.

- *Reverencing the culture* refers to how nurses must respect the values and norms of those with whom they partner.

- *Refraining from harm* refers to following recommendations from leading authorities such as WHO for care that is not harmful.

- *Reducing the biomedical and ethnocentricity threat* refers to the need to be mindful of the positive and negative consequences of introducing Western biomedical treatments into a culture that is reluctant to accept the change.

Additionally, Crump and Sugarman (2010) created a work group, Working Group on Ethics Guidelines for Global Health Training (WEIGHT), to develop guidelines for the leaders of health professional training programs that occur in international settings. We recommend that our readers look at this publication to see the full set of guidelines, but the key issues focus upon attainment of mutually beneficial goals, the development of long-term partnerships with short-term experiences nested within them, the careful selection and preparation of trainees for the experience, the efforts to achieve cultural sensitivity, the respect of ethical issues in licensing and patient information, the consideration of the local needs as priorities, and the importance of sustainability of programs.

One of Crigger and Holcomb's (2007) recommendations that we emphasize throughout the book is the importance of culture. In the sidebar earlier in the chapter, we noted that Diane Martins entered a culture different from her own when she began her work with a homeless population, indicating diversity exists within local communities as well as across international borders. Responsible service requires attention to culture and diversity. Nurses report that immersion into another culture increases cultural competence for the nurse (Wood & Atkins, 2006; Waite & Calamaro, 2010), but we believe that nurses must prepare for volunteer service with as much knowledge and attention to cultural diversity issues as they do for all other aspects of preparation. Educational and practice settings cite cultural competence as a goal for nursing. We believe that *cultural competence* is a process rather than an outcome that anyone can achieve for a culture that is not their own. Many models of cultural competence are available for nurses (Duke, Connor, & McEldowney, 2009), and we offer references for them in Appendix A, "Resources." Likewise, the term *cultural safety* emerged from work in New Zealand to ensure safe care for the indigenous Maori population (Duke et al., 2009). We consider cultural competence and cultural safety as goals for nurses to provide appropriate care for the diversity within populations that they serve.

Some who have written about the nurse volunteer situation use terms such as *cultural awareness*, the exploration of one's own cultural background; *cultural desire*, the energy that moves nurses to seek to become culturally competent

(Campinha-Bacote, 2005); and *cultural sensitivity* or the identification of one's assumptions of one's social and personal background that affect one's perspective on culture (Duke et al., 2009). We prefer to use the term *cultural humility* for the work of nurse volunteers. Cultural humility is a process of reflection and critique of one's self to identify biases and beliefs. Such humility enables nurses to meet others as equals by reducing power differences when they deal with patient- or community-focused interviews or approaches to care (Foster, 2009; Tervalon & Murray-Garcia, 1998). This process where nurse volunteers move beyond sensitivity to differences and toward being responsible for interactions with others helps them to learn about those with whom they work without stereotyping or using dominant biomedical models as universal standards (Levi, 2009).

To learn more about cultural competence and other strategies that promote appropriate care for diverse populations, we suggest that you consult some of the resources we offer in Appendix A, particularly the National Center for Cultural Competence at Georgetown University (http://nccc.georgetown.edu); the Cross Cultural Health Care Program (http://www.xculture.org/about.php); the Health Resources and Services Administration (HRSA), available at http://www.hrsa.gov/culturalcompetence/; and the Stanford University Center for Biomedical Ethics film series, *Worlds Apart*, available at http://medethicsfilms.stanford.edu/worldsapart/.

Throughout the book we integrate issues that we believe are essential for nurses to understand to provide ethical and responsible care for those they serve. Nurses must also incorporate the recommendations of Crigger and Holcomb (2007) and Crump and Sugarman (2010) into their work. The needs are great and nurses are well suited to meet the needs and to address the injustice of health inequalities. In the words of Martin Luther King, Jr., from the Letter from Birmingham Jail, 1963, "Injustice anywhere is a threat to justice everywhere."

BECOMING AN EFFECTIVE VOLUNTEER

- Learn from those nurses who preceded us as volunteers.

- Read about nurse volunteers of today in settings at home and abroad.

- Consider the community where you will volunteer to identify its strengths and needs.

- Read about nurses Claire Bertschinger, Greg Mortenson, and the late Lillian Carter, who began as volunteers but whose work now impacts the lives of many throughout the world.

- Consider the impact of globalization upon health.

- Consult the resources in Appendix A to learn more about global issues.

- Use the Millennium Development Goals as a guide for planning volunteer projects.

- Remember the environment and the impact volunteer projects can have to improve environmental sustainability.

- Consult resources for environmental health such as www.envirn.org and www.noharm.org.

- Consider the ethical implications of your volunteer work.

- Learn about culture. Review some of the resources that address how to respect culture in nursing and health care.

CHAPTER 2

THINKING SERIOUSLY ABOUT VOLUNTEERING

Volunteering can be rewarding and in many instances a life-changing experience for the nurse who takes advantage of a call to serve as a volunteer. As caring professionals, nurses commonly respond to opportunities to serve others in local or distant settings.

Possibly, you have long dreamed of serving others in a distant country or have heard about a volunteer opportunity you would like to explore. To make effective decisions about whether volunteering is best for you and to find the right program to fit your needs, you should first complete a self-assessment inventory tool in step-wise sequence, locate likely programs or opportunities that fit your needs, and ensure a good fit between your skills and your preferred program. In this chapter we provide you with assessment questions for you to complete your personal self-assessment. The volunteering situation might be just what you are seeking, or it might not be right for you.

Nurses have a variety of skills and interests, and a volunteer assignment might not be right for everyone. The most important step before making any commitment to volunteer is to complete your own self-assessment. You need to consider personal, social, and professional issues in order to determine if volunteering is a good fit for you. Understanding these issues will help you determine how effective you can be as a nurse volunteer. In this chapter we offer you a self-assessment inventory tool for you to complete in step-wise sequence.

PERSONAL ISSUES

Assessment of your own personal issues is the most important aspect of your self-assessment. Only you can determine what motivates you to volunteer, what your interests are in serving in a particular location or with a particular population, and what work brings you personal satisfaction. We invite you to really explore what is your passion, what gives you energy, and what motivates you to consider becoming a volunteer or extending your service into new areas.

MOTIVATION

If you can identify what you feel passionate about, then you can begin to understand what motivates you to volunteer. Begin by making a list of those things that you find make you happy, give you energy, and keep you engaged. Some of those passions might be useful in your volunteer role. For example, maybe you are a nurse who works with adults, but you love to spend time with children. You might find that the joy of seeing children happy and smiling because of your volunteer efforts can brighten any discouraging day. Possibly, you love music and play the guitar. Music might add to the volunteer program, might relax you in the evening, or might create camaraderie among volunteers. Or you might have a special compassion for those with physical impairments or for older adults. Your talents and interests are essential attributes that define you as a volunteer. Identifying your passion can help you plan for how you might enjoy those passions in the volunteer setting. Working with what you find you are most passionate about can add meaning to the volunteer setting.

Next, you need to think about what has led you to consider volunteering. Many nurses would respond, "I want to give back to society." You might have spent years dreaming of using your nursing skills to help others in overseas communities. For example, you might have felt a deep call to offer your services in response to seeing news of a disaster such as the Asian tsunami of 2004, Hurricane Katrina in 2005, or the devastating earthquake in Haiti in 2010. After the earthquake in Port-au-Prince, Haiti, on January 12, 2010, a tremendous outpouring of support came from nurses in many countries. Within days of the disaster, thousands of emergency department, surgical, and critical care nurses, and even those in other specialties, registered with organizations to offer their nursing services. Some of the critical care nurses who responded at the time of the earthquake not only traveled to Haiti in the weeks following but have also returned for extended stays during the first 6 months post-disaster and made commitments for continued service there (Regena Deck, personal communication, January 4, 2011).

Some nurses who have given years of service to people in need in their own communities have a desire to venture further from home for new experiences. For example, Jeanne spent 7 years volunteering at a center for immigrants and refugees where she met people from all over the world who had immigrated to the Providence, Rhode Island, area. Volunteering in the Dominican Republic, Guatemala, and Haiti, where many of the immigrants came from, provided wonderful opportunities for her to learn more about their culture, their health practices, and the issues they faced as immigrants to the United States.

For some, the motivation to volunteer develops from religious faith or community service organization mission and values. For others, the desire to volunteer grows out of a strong belief in social justice. Nurses who have worked with the group Doctors for Global Health indicate that their commitment to social justice, a core ethical value for the nursing profession, led them to seek a group that promotes social justice in their mission and values (Myers, 2010).

Jack Geiger notes in his keynote speech for the 2002 assembly for Doctors for Global Health that health care professionals do the work to improve local and global health for three reasons. He states:

> The real message in our volunteer work and in our human rights work is threefold: What we are saying to the people we work with is that their lives are as worthy as our own…that by our presence and our work we demonstrate a commitment to the idea of equity…for the lives of the people we work with. Second, our work goes, beyond our medical tasks of prevention and cure… in the principles of working with the community…

empowering people and communities. The third thing we are really doing is saying to people we work with that, we presume there will be a future. We presume social change. We presume a future that will be different. (Geiger, 2010)

You might agree with his comments and believe that your motivations match what he describes. However, you might also find that your reasons to consider this work are different. Take a few minutes and write yourself a short personal letter explaining what you feel is your motivation and from where the desire to serve originated.

If you have just begun to think more seriously about taking on a volunteer role, you might have heard stories from a friend or colleague that motivated you to consider volunteering at this time. Possibly, you want to learn about another culture, or you are fascinated by the exotic image you have of a particular distant country. Maybe a news documentary caught your interest. You might also simply desire to travel and are looking for opportunities to do so. Look at the questions in Table 2.1 to see if you can identify your motivations to volunteer overseas.

TABLE 2.1

SELF-ASSESSMENT INVENTORY: MOTIVATION FOR SERVICE
How did I become interested in global health and nursing?
In what ways have I put my concern for others into action?
What have been the experiences in my life that might have influenced this interest?
Do I have a strong desire to travel to one particular setting?
Am I seeking adventure in a volunteer assignment?

TABLE 2.1, continued

SELF-ASSESSMENT INVENTORY: MOTIVATION FOR SERVICE

Am I seeking excitement and change in my life?

Did a friend encourage me to join in the same volunteer assignment?

Am I seeking the opportunity to learn more about another culture?

Does my religious faith motivate me to volunteer?

Am I trying to get away from problems at home?

Has a recent media message inspired my desire to serve in a disaster?

What do I think I can contribute?

Do I believe that I can save people who live in poverty by my volunteer efforts?

If you are honest in assessing your motivations, you must also consider if you are possibly looking to find some exciting change in your life because of boredom with a job or a life upheaval event, such as the end of a relationship. It's important to recognize such issues because volunteer work is challenging and should not be undertaken as an escape from personal challenges. In addition, if your motivation is to convert others to your faith, or if you believe you can save others from lives of poverty, you will not be an effective volunteer. Throughout the book we emphasize that volunteering is a partnership where volunteers are guests in the host country, and, as guests, should not impose their own cultural and religious beliefs upon those they come to serve.

This honest appraisal of your motivations will provide you with a better understanding of yourself, making you better prepared if challenges arise in the volunteer setting. Also, after you understand what motivates you, you might discover that a study-abroad or language-immersion experience is a better fit for an interest about learning a new language or learning about another culture. If you realize you are seeking an adventure, you might instead seek an adventure travel option.

COMMITMENT

A second important issue for you to consider is how much time you have to give at this point in your life. If you are working full-time and have family responsibilities, volunteering close to home in your own community might be the best situation for you. On the other hand, if you are employed part-time or are semi-retired from active nursing, you might feel you can devote more time to pursue your passion for service. Some nurses who volunteer overseas on a yearly basis elect to work as permanent float pool nursing staff so they can obtain time off to do volunteer work. Many nurse educators are willing to volunteer during school breaks, during the summer months, or during a sabbatical leave.

If you only have 1 week, then your volunteer experience will be very different than if you have a month or more to spend in the volunteer setting. Though more time in a volunteer setting offers you a richer experience in which you are more likely to learn about the culture and collaborate to improve health, nurses acknowledge that even 1-week experiences can be rewarding and life changing. To plan for how much time you can commit to a volunteer assignment, ask yourself the questions in Table 2.2.

TABLE 2.2

SELF-ASSESSMENT INVENTORY: TIME COMMITMENT

How much time am I able to commit to volunteer work?

Am I seeking a one-time experience or do I hope to continue this type of service?

Am I looking for intermittent service (such as once a year for 2 weeks)?

Do I want long term (2–6 months stay) service?

How much time am I able to take off from work?

Does my employer support such volunteer service?

Could I take time to volunteer without using all my vacation?

PERSONAL RESPONSIBILITIES

What about your personal responsibilities? If you have home responsibilities that cannot easily be delegated to someone else, it might not be feasible for you to travel. If you are caring for family members or have relatives who are seriously ill, it might not be the best time to travel a great distance. Ask yourself if you can take time away from being a caretaker for dependents such as disabled or minor children or elderly relatives. Evaluate if you can be away from other personal responsibilities. Frequently parents of young children make service trips to distant countries and are unprepared for how profoundly they miss their family. Prompt communication with family is difficult at best, and if you plan to be away while a family member is ill or needs your help or advice, it might not be the right time for you to make such a trip.

LOCATION

Do you have a particular place that you have always wanted to visit for a variety of reasons? Many nurses were Peace

Corps volunteers in their early adult years, some even before they entered a nursing education program. After spending up to 3 years in a country in their youth, they desire to return as short-term volunteers. Such knowledge of a particular country and its culture can be a strong motivation for nurses to want to return and participate in other volunteer experiences in that country. While we may have some sort of vision of what we might find in a place that has captured our interest, we need to also consider what might be some of the positive surprises, but also the challenges, we may encounter. In the sidebar below, Pamela Llewellyn (personal communication, 2011) of the United Kingdom offers some thoughts about location when volunteering.

CHANGING LIVES

How important is the location of a volunteer placement abroad? When I began to tell people that I had applied to become a Voluntary Service Overseas (VSO) volunteer, I was asked, "Where would you like to go?" On my application form I had said somewhere warm rather than cold and in a community rather than isolated, but otherwise I was open to what I was offered. I felt passive in the selection process. Mongolia was discussed briefly, but I felt 6 months below freezing would not suit my chilblains or my need for company.

When I was offered Uganda, I e-mailed existing volunteers, looked at maps, found a travel book, and looked on the Volzone website. First of all I considered the placement outline (job description) and then moved on to the location and setting. Masindi is "up country" but a busy town, and there are other volunteers. Uganda is an 8-hour flight from the U.K., Masindi a 4-hour bus journey from Kampala, and the average annual temperature is a mere 78 degrees Fahrenheit. It seemed to tick most of the boxes on my checklist, and I decided to accept.

I have been here nearly 4 months. Cultural and professional shock lessens with continual exposure, but some day-to-day challenges remain. The travel book, the map, and the Volzone information did not lie, but if I look at these now I see something different than before I came here. This corner of Uganda is a harsh environment and very poor. The majority of its people are subsistence farmers, scratching a living off a small plot of land near their hand-built homes. Investment and development here are low. Roads leading out of Masindi are not paved, so travel along the compacted marram is slow and uncomfortable. In dry weather, the roads send up a continual blanket of orange dust; after rain, the ruts become deeper and sometimes flood. Just to the north is the entrance to one of the country's largest national parks, Murchison Falls, but beyond this up to the Congo and Sudanese borders are vast areas of conflict and are out of bounds to VSO volunteers.

I have recently moved around the country visiting other VSO placements. Each location has its own challenges and advantages. I have stayed in a house with no inside water or toilet, but the BBC World Service reception was constant and clear, a real joy! Paved roads in the southwest bring ease of travel, accessibility, delivery of goods and services, fewer punctures, and less dust. Most volunteers spend some time travelling, and they need areas of natural beauty to gladden the eyes and the heart when thousands of miles from home. There is a lot to consider about a placement location, but like me you may not discover reality until you arrive.

Other nurses have worked with a particular immigrant population in their own home community. Still other nurses seek to travel to a country close to their home. For example, many nurses in the United States travel to Haiti or the Dominican Republic to volunteer because of proximity and short flights. For nurses around the world, the ability to travel on a non-stop flight to the volunteer destination makes travel and expenses more feasible.

PHYSICAL DEMANDS OF VOLUNTEER SERVICE

Physical stamina is necessary for most volunteer assignments. In many areas, nurses must walk distances on rugged terrain, often carrying supplies and their personal water for the day. In many programs, volunteers must travel in the back of trucks, climb into and out of the vehicle, and stand or sit uncomfortably in the back for long rides on bumpy roads. Though some locations provide food and water as part of the cost to the volunteer, others require that volunteers participate in the procurement and preparation of food for the group. Again, this means that the volunteer might have to walk into the town or city to purchase food and supplies. The time needed to complete chores in the living setting adds to what is often a long day of volunteer work.

Many assignments are located in tropical climates where the temperatures are quite warm and air conditioning is uncommon. You have to tolerate the heat with no air conditioning both in housing and clinical settings. Most housing for nurse volunteers is in non air-conditioned settings. Thousands of volunteers in Haiti after the 2010 earthquake stayed in tents. In other settings, volunteers stay in dorms or bunkhouses. Together, we have stayed in a wide range of settings. Jeanne, for example, has stayed in housing that includes bunk rooms of 13–18 people with only about 18 inches between beds and limited space for personal belongings, in a small dormitory room in a church-run dorm facility, in a semi-private room in a small home on the grounds of the volunteer site, and in a small apartment at a guest house during a long-term stay in Uganda. In each of these settings, bottled water was necessary, showers were often cold or had to be bucket showers, mosquito nets were necessary, and the typical comforts of home were distinctly lacking. Typically, there are few or no small appliances, television, telephones, or access to a computer.

Occasionally, a volunteer program houses the volunteers with families or in a hotel. To stay with families, the volunteer should be somewhat fluent in the language to make the stay easier. In addition, food and water are a concern as they might not be prepared with the same standards as at home. However, the opportunity to learn more about the culture and make lasting friendships with local people far outweighs any challenges a volunteer might encounter.

Hotel accommodations provide the opportunity for comfortable housing, and needed rest, yet many volunteers find that living in a hotel where the comforts far exceed those of the local people creates emotional conflict and a constant reminder of the poverty the locals face daily. Most volunteer nurses prefer to have accommodations more congruent with the housing of the people they serve rather than undergo a reimmersion into the local community every day.

If you elect to volunteer outside your country, learn about the living conditions for volunteers and honestly assess if you can deal with them. Many first-time volunteers become upset by the lack of hot showers, flush toilets, clean floors, or personal space. Others are afraid of insects or other animals nearby. Though some volunteers adjust to these issues within a few days, others are uncomfortable and unhappy during the entire stay because of the living conditions.

Also, before you embark on a volunteer assignment, get to know the daily schedule and determine if you can handle the physical demands. You might routinely take naps during the day or require a great deal of rest to manage long working hours. You may be a light sleeper who cannot tolerate being awakened nightly by roosters crowing, by dogs barking, or even by motorized corn grinders run by women who begin their work at 3 a.m. During the day hours, you might not have an opportunity to rest until dinnertime. Thus, it's important to be mindful of your physical limits.

EMOTIONAL CONCERNS

The desire to serve others can be highly motivating and offer great joy and gratitude. After you are in the field, however, the poverty and tragedy of human life can be emotionally draining. In some settings, nurses see children die on a daily basis or hear stories from those they work with about their poverty and hunger. In these instances, nursing and medical care alone cannot improve their lives. Only structural changes to the economic, political, and social aspects of their lives can bring safe food and water, shelter, and necessities. For many nurses, the sense of being helpless to make sustaining change for the people they serve can be troubling.

Additionally, those who travel overseas have to face the emotional adjustments to being in a new country. For many nurses, being in a country where the language is not one's own or where the nurse is in the minority is a new experience. Many nurses, particularly young nurses or nursing students, become homesick or feel uncomfortable in unknown surroundings. The political climate might be vastly different. Some nurses have been alarmed to see guards holding rifles along the road or in public buildings. In some countries, you have to pass frequent military checkpoints. Accordingly, you need to be prepared for the differences in the politics and culture of where you are planning to volunteer. In future chapters we explain more about how to prepare for the social, political, and cultural differences you might experience overseas.

SOCIAL ISSUES

In Chapter 1, we spoke about some of the cultural issues that might affect you personally. To assess your own needs, you must consider some of the social issues that will affect you. Living in a new environment offers great opportunity to learn about other cultures. You will find it very rewarding to make new friends in another country. Often, if nurses return to the same volunteer program, they watch children grow, keep relationships with local people, and enjoy the rewards of learning about a new community. Julia maintains contact with nurses in Rwanda and Ethiopia that she has known for decades. At the same time, however, as a guest in the community, you must be aware of cultural differences so as not to offend your hosts.

Also, to get the most benefit from working overseas, or in a community whose language differs from your own, you must consider your ability to communicate in that language. Jeanne had studied Latin and French while in school but had no Spanish language skills when she planned to travel to Guatemala. In preparation for that volunteer experience, she took Spanish language lessons. Though her Spanish skills are still intermediate, she can communicate with most people in countries where Spanish is spoken. Though not all nurse volunteers can become fluent in a new language, the availability of skilled medical interpreters, preferably from the host country, can make a great difference for communication in the volunteer setting.

Another question to consider: How important is it for you to feel integrated into the community you are serving? As we mentioned earlier in the chapter, some programs house volunteers away from the people they work with, and volunteers feel disconnected from the local hosts. This is particularly true of those who stay in hotels and not in the community itself. All leisure time is spent with the team members, which allows for no interaction with the people there. For other nurses, this separation is a much-needed break from their immersion into a new culture.

This point raises other issues of privacy and personal space. Most volunteer settings offer little personal space for volunteers. In many places, the sleeping quarters are bunkhouses where 4 to 20 people share a room. Communal living areas for relaxation might be small and shared by as many as 35 people. Often these are outdoors and in case of rain offer no private personal or quiet space. You need to recognize that if you are someone who likes quiet time alone, you might find this impossible during your volunteer stay. Living and working among other volunteers who you have only just met offer opportunities for new friendships, but can require challenging adjustments as well.

PROFESSIONAL ISSUES

As nurses, we bring a variety of skills and experience to a volunteer experience. Some have public health nursing experience and skills. Others have critical care skills, acute care skills, or specific expertise in areas such as diabetes management or neonatal high-risk care. To consider the best match between your professional skills and experience and the program that you elect to volunteer with, you must make a thorough assessment of your professional expertise (see Table 2.3). First, determine your scope of practice. If you are an RN or an LPN, then you must work within the appropriate practice standards. Likewise, if you hold advanced practice certification, as a nurse practitioner, for example, you must only practice in the area of your certification. Within your practice scope, you then need to identify your specialty skills. For example, if you are skilled in health assessment, you might be very effective in primary care, or possibly you have knowledge of tropical diseases because you work in a travel clinic. If you work as a surgical nurse, you might want to travel with a multidisciplinary surgical team. As volunteers, we must offer those we work with the same standard of expertise that we offer our patients in our home country.

TABLE 2.3

SELF-ASSESSMENT INVENTORY: CLINICAL EXPERTISE

CLINICAL NURSING EXPERTISE	*RATING*
Medical nursing	
Medical subspecialty, such as hemodialysis, burns, etc.	
Surgical nursing	
Surgical subspecialty, such as orthopedics	
Critical care	
Women's health, and perinatal health	
Children's health	
Mental health	
Population and public health	
Advanced practice	
Specialty role (diabetes educator, wound specialist, etc.)	
Other noteworthy clinical practice	

Beyond your clinical specialty are other skills that can make you a better volunteer. The assessment of these skills helps you determine what role is the best fit for your volunteer work. Look at the following checklist (Table 2.4) and assess which skills describe your strengths. For example, how strong are your communication skills? The ability to communicate with other volunteers and with interpreters or host partners is essential to successful programs. Are you a leader? Leadership skills are important to volunteer settings. The ability to create successful partnerships is improved with nurse leadership skills. Are you a nursing educator in a clinic or academic setting? Expertise in curriculum development, teaching and learning strategies, assessment, and evaluation are needed in many settings where nurses work with nurse colleagues in the host setting. Empowering nurses and health care workers (sometimes village health workers) is important to building a more effective health care system to promote health in limited resource settings.

TABLE 2.4

SELF-ASSESSMENT INVENTORY: PROFESSIONAL SKILLS

SKILL	RATING
Oral communication	
Written communication	
Leadership	
Assessment and planning	
Curriculum development	
Program evaluation	
Community engagement	

NEXT STEPS

After you have completed a thorough self-assessment, you should have a good profile of what you are seeking from a volunteer assignment—and more importantly a profile of what you have to offer to a program. We cannot emphasize enough that this process requires a great deal of time and thought if you want it to result in a thorough and honest assessment of your motivation, talents, skills, strengths, and limitations. After this important step is completed, you can move on to the following chapters in which we guide you to match your profile to a program to ensure a good fit, to select an appropriate volunteer opportunity, and then begin the preparation in order to make a successful trip.

BECOMING AN EFFECTIVE VOLUNTEER

- Assess your motivation to volunteer.
- Think about the commitment you can make.
- Consider your personal responsibilities.
- Think about location to anticipate the volunteer setting.
- Evaluate your physical stamina and emotional responses.
- Consider social and cultural issues.
- Identify your professional expertise.
- Assess other important nursing skill sets.
- Complete your self assessment.

CHAPTER 3

FINDING A VOLUNTEER PROGRAM

In this chapter we explore important factors about programs and organizations where you might find your ideal volunteering opportunity. We also discuss how nurses are likely to learn about volunteer opportunities and some of the advantages and disadvantages of each source of information and ask you to consider what you are looking for in a program. We offer information on some of the common volunteer roles that nurses assume in direct care for people, as consultants, and as nurse educators and address important issues for you to consider in looking into specific programs or organizations. Finally, we give examples of organizations and nursing service roles.

Most nurses serve as volunteers with a particular program or organization. Exceptions to this are nurses who volunteer while living in another country with a family member or other person. In these cases nurses have been able to develop partnering relationships with local programs abroad. Julia served as a nurse volunteer in Turkey while she and her family lived there for 1 year during a sabbatical, but this situation is unusual.

Many nurses volunteer with a program local to their own home or work environment, having learned about it through local nursing colleagues. Jeanne's first trip as a volunteer nurse to Guatemala was with a project connected with Brown University at the time she was in graduate school there. She was able to speak directly with medical and nursing volunteers who had spent time in the host location and learn about the role she might have as a volunteer. Despite preparation, taking a conversational-Spanish class, and learning from the experienced volunteers, she still encountered many unexpected situations as a first time volunteer nurse. This experience then guided her about what she needed to learn about the next volunteer opportunity. She then spent a great deal of time speaking personally or by telephone to nurses who had volunteered with the new organization she selected. In addition, she sought information about other similar opportunities to compare various program factors. From this careful comparison, she felt better prepared for the next volunteer experience. We cannot emphasize enough the importance of spending sufficient time learning about the organization and the expected nurse volunteer role. We speak to this point throughout the chapter.

Jeanne's experience with a locally based program is similar to those of many of our colleagues who have shared their stories with us over the years. The majority of nurse volunteers find the program where they volunteer through local networks—friends, colleagues at work, hospital-sponsored programs, or local church and civic groups. This offers you the advantage of having experienced volunteers nearby to talk to about the program. Yet, the actual program role for the nurse might not be the best fit for the volunteer. So, how can you find the best program or organization where you can share your skills? We recommend learning about a variety of programs and organizations before you commit to serve as a volunteer.

WHERE NURSES OFTEN FIND VOLUNTEER PROGRAMS OR ORGANIZATIONS

Nurses often ask us where they can locate volunteer opportunities. Volunteer opportunities in your local community are often well advertised through the media and social contacts in your own community. For those of you considering volunteer opportunities some distance from home in your own or another country, we discuss how you can locate programs through your own local networks, from nursing publications, from professional nursing organizations, through the Internet and from published volunteer guidebooks. These sources can also provide ideas for those nurses who are looking for ideas in their local areas as well.

LOCAL NETWORKS

First, consider those programs that you hear about from local networks or word-of-mouth. The first-hand accounts from local volunteers can provide you with opportunities to develop a better vision of what the volunteer role might be. However, it is important to learn about other programs that might be a better fit for your skills. We offer some suggestions about specific programs in Appendix B to help you learn more about various programs and organizations and how to locate them. Matching the self-assessment that you completed in Chapter 2 with the right program means matching your skills to the program that best fits you. We talk more about how to match your profile to the organization that best fits you in Chapter 4.

NURSING PUBLICATIONS

A second route to learn about programs is through nursing publications. Increasingly, nurses publish reports about their personal experiences with volunteer programs (see Box 3.1).

Nurses also publish examples of volunteer service in specialty journals such as

- *Public Health Nursing* (O'Hara, 2006)
- *Journal of Nursing Education* (Evanson & Zust, 2006)
- *Journal of Continuing Education in Nursing* (Bosworth et al., 2006)
- *Nurse Educator* (Kollar & Ailinger, 2002)
- *Journal of Cultural Diversity* (Patsdaughter, Christensen, Kelley, Masters, & Ndiwane, 2001)
- *Journal of Multicultural Nursing and Health*
- *Journal of Transcultural Nursing* (Riner & Becklenberg, 2001)

- *Nursing and Health Care Perspectives* (Jarrett, Hummel, & Whitney, 2005; Ailinger, & Carty, 1996)

- *Journal of Professional Nursing* (Callister & Hobbins-Garbett, 2000)

- *Reflections on Nursing Leadership* (Baran, 2010; Cavanaugh-Sutkus, 2008; Nash, 2008; Watson, 2010)

The advantage of published information is that you learn about the specific experience of the nurse author and the nursing role assumed in that volunteer setting. Many authors welcome questions from readers seeking more information and publish their contact information, or can be found easily online. Personal communication is not always possible or available, but is worth investigating in case it is.

NURSING PROFESSIONAL ORGANIZATIONS

Many nursing organizations can be an excellent source of information. For example, the Association of Community Health Nursing Educators (ACHNE) holds an annual meeting where many nurses present papers or posters about their global health experiences. Other examples are the American College of Nurse-Midwives, which has a Department of Global Outreach (http://www.midwife.org/global.cfm); the National Association of Pediatric Nurse Practitioners, which has a special interest group dedicated to global health (http://www.napnap.org/aboutUs/SpecialInterestGroups/GlobalHealthCare.aspx); and the Oncology Nursing Society with its special interest group, Transcultural Nursing Issues its http://transcultural.vc.ons.org/). In addition, the Association of periOperative Registered Nurses (AORN) hosts a global perspectives column in its journal. These are a few of the examples of specialty organizations that focus upon global health. Also, an alliance of nurses called the Global Alliance for Nursing and Midwifery hosts a Listserv that is a great resource for nurses interested in global health (http://my.ibpinitiative. org/ganm).

INTERNET RESOURCES

Many nurses find their volunteer opportunities through Internet research. This can be useful as a way both to broaden your knowledge of what types of programs are available and also to learn about the organization, its mission and goals, and past successes. The advantage of Internet resources is that they are readily available and are usually updated on a regular basis, enabling you to explore a variety of opportunities anonymously and rapidly to determine what might interest you before you make any direct contact with an organization. The disadvantage is that you do not have immediate personal contact with the leaders of the program or organization. Frequently, the nurse's role is not clearly defined on the Internet website, and you must take the time to make direct contact with a personal representative to learn more.

PUBLISHED VOLUNTEER GUIDE BOOKS

Several volunteer guidebooks have been published that might be useful for nursing volunteers. These include *Volunteering: The Selfish Benefits: Achieve Deep-Down Satisfaction and Create Desire in Others* (Bennett, 2001), *A Practical Guide to Global Health Service* (O'Neil, 2006), *Volunteering Around the Globe: Life-Changing Travel Adventures* (Stone & Jones, 2008), and *How to Live Your Dream of Volunteering*

Overseas (Collins, DeZerega, & Heckscher, 2002). Each of these references offers suggestions for potential volunteers, and most also list a number of volunteer opportunities. The advantages offered by these books are the extensive experience of the authors, the practical suggestions they offer, and the listings of possible volunteer opportunities. You might elect to consult them as a supplement to what we offer in this resource. The disadvantage is that these references address neither the specific needs of the nurse volunteer nor the particular issues of nursing volunteer roles.

WHAT YOU NEED TO CONSIDER IN SELECTING A PROGRAM OR ORGANIZATION

The following discussion of organizational issues related to specific volunteer programs can serve as a guide for you as you learn about volunteer opportunities. We address issues such as the philosophy and history of the program, nursing role, focus of nursing interventions, location for volunteer service, expenses, and what the organization provides to meet personal needs. We offer a table (see Table 3.1) to help you organize these issues for each program that you investigate. Organizations often provide materials that are helpful for the volunteer, such as *Working with Humanitarian Organisations: A Guide for Nurses, Midwives, and Health Care Professionals* (Medecins Sans Frontieres et al., 2010), *Global Standards for the Initial Education of Professional Nurses and Midwives*, (WHO, 2009), *A Core Competency Framework for International Health Consultants* (World Health Professional Alliance, 2007), and *A Guide to Volunteering Overseas* (Health Volunteers Overseas, 2007).

TABLE 3.1

ORGANIZATIONAL FACTORS

CLINICAL NURSING EXPERTISE RATING								
NAME OF PROGRAM OR ORGANIZATION	MISSION, GOALS AND VALUES	HISTORY	NURSE ROLE	FOCUS OF NURSING INTERVENTION	LOCATION	EXPENSES	PERSONAL NEEDS

PHILOSOPHY OF THE PROGRAM

The most important question you need to ask about a potential volunteer opportunity is the philosophy of the program. Every organization should have a mission, vision, values, and goals that can help you to identify how its mission fits with your own goals for volunteering. When Jeanne sought a more long-term volunteer experience during a sabbatical leave from her faculty position, she investigated a variety of programs and organizations. She applied to Health Volunteers Overseas (HVO) because the mission was congruent with her belief in partnership and empowerment. (See Box 3.1 to see the HVO mission, vision, and values.)

BOX 3.1

HEALTH VOLUNTEERS OVERSEAS—MISSION, VISION, AND VALUES

MISSION STATEMENT

Health Volunteers Overseas (www.hvousa.org) is a private non-profit organization dedicated to improving the availability and quality of health care in developing countries through the training and education of local health care providers.

VISION

HVO will be recognized as a global leader in the development and implementation of educational programs designed to empower health care providers in developing countries.

GUIDING PRINCIPLES

HVO programs will be staffed by highly qualified health care professionals who will demonstrate the highest standards of professional and personal conduct. Sensitivity and respect for the cultural and social beliefs and practices of the host country should guide professional and personal behavior.

Programs will vary according to the needs of the countries and the educational priorities identified. However, there are certain principles that apply across all programs:

- *Training will focus on local diseases and health conditions;*

- *Practices, procedures, and skills taught will be both relevant and realistic and should include, when appropriate, a focus on prevention;*

- *Programs will promote lifelong learning;*

- *Whenever possible, programs will focus on training local personnel who will assume the roles of both educator and provider.*

Volunteers are encouraged to make maximum use of locally available equipment and supplies in order to foster long-term sustainability. If donations of equipment, medications, or other supplies are deemed essential to accomplish the educational goals of the project, these donations should be appropriate to the needs of the site and meet international donation standards as established by WHO or other similar organizations.

CORE VALUES

Health Volunteers Overseas:

- *Programs will promote lifelong learning;*

- *Implements innovative, effective programs that meet the needs of the host country and institution, are sustainable, and build local capacity.*

- *Recruits qualified, committed, culturally sensitive health care professionals as volunteers.*

> - *Works in partnership with other organizations, host governments and institutions, and local health care professionals in a spirit of mutual respect and cooperation.*
> - *Is dedicated to good stewardship and lifelong learning (HVO, 2010a).*

Other programs have been developed through various faith communities to provide service in areas of need. Though many do accept volunteers who are not members of the particular faith community, you need to learn as much as you can about their philosophy and religious perspective. You might find that the philosophy of the program includes a religious perspective that is congruent with or differs from your own.

HISTORY AND OPERATIONAL MANAGEMENT OF THE ORGANIZATION

You can identify important issues about an organization when you learn about its history. You will want to know how long the organization has existed and how it has grown over time. It will be important to learn how nurses have been involved with the organization over the years as well. Further, you will want to know how the organization sustains its program both financially and through human resources. You must learn about how the organization partners with host community members to measure how well the organization meets the needs of those living in the host country. Identify if the organization does any program evaluation for program improvement.

A sign of a healthy organization is the type of information it seeks from volunteers. No nurse should travel to another country and plan to practice nursing without some documentation of licensure and/or certification. Always remember that we are guests in the host country and should have the permission of the host country Ministry of Health or similar governing body to legalize our practice. We say more about some of the ethical and legal aspects of nursing practice in other countries in Chapter 8. In addition, most organizations require a copy of your nursing degree or diploma and recommendations that speak to your nursing skills and personal character, and some even require fingerprints and criminal background checks. These requirements should not be deterrents to your work, but rather indicate a sound organization that shows respect to the health system of the host country.

WHAT TYPE OF ROLE MIGHT I EXPECT IN MY VOLUNTEER SERVICE?

We cannot say enough about the importance of investigating the role expectations of the program or organization where you elect to volunteer. As discussed in Chapter 2, nurses have a variety of professional skills and particular expertise according to practice and education. To make the best fit between your particular expertise and the organizational needs, you need to learn what the expected role might be. For example, those nurses who travel to the Dominican Republic with Intercultural Nursing, Inc., can expect to be involved in daily clinics where they use their nursing expertise with individual patients. Some educational opportunities exist, but the majority of the work is direct care. In contrast, HVO is an organization whose focus is on partnering with host country health professionals to advance their knowledge and skills in specific specialty areas. Nurses who volunteer with this organization can expect to spend time educating other nurses, either in a classroom or clinical setting. Though they might have contact with patients, the role is not to provide direct care but rather to serve as an educator.

SOME COMMON VOLUNTEER ROLES

Our profession requires specialized knowledge and skills for professional practice (ANA, 2010), and we use our expertise in a variety of roles in settings where we volunteer. Our professional role expectations include the following:

- Nurse as provider of direct care to the sick
- Nurse as designer, coordinator, and manager of care
- Nurse as patient educator
- Nurse as translator of knowledge to patients
- Nurse as collaborator with the health care team
- Nurse as supervisor of those to whom care is delegated
- Nurse as patient advocate
- Nurse as monitor of outcomes

The essential knowledge and skills of the baccalaureate-prepared professional nurse include the ability for comprehensive assessment of individuals, sound clinical judgment and decision making, participatory decision making, health promotion and clinical prevention, population health, organizational leadership, and ability to monitor outcomes and evaluate care (AACN, 2008; ANA, 2010). Though practice standards vary across nations, nurse volunteers must abide by the standards of practice for their own country.

TABLE 3.2

EXAMPLES OF NURSING INTERVENTIONS IN VOLUNTEER ROLES

FOCUS OF INTERVENTION	NURSING EXAMPLE	CHARACTERISTICS	DESIRED OUTCOME	REQUISITE NURSING SKILLS
Individual	Manuela Sanchez	Individual cared for by a volunteer nurse visiting from another country at a community clinic in Latin America	Improved health for Manuela or improved capacity for self-care	Individual nursing assessment Health teaching for self-care Treatment plan and medication administration Evidence-based nursing interventions Referral for health care needs
Community	Small town in Uganda	Community has high incidence of infant mortality at a location 2 hours from hospital	Partnership development for community-based participatory research to reduce infant mortality	Community assessment Communication skills Community engagement Cultural humility

FOCUS OF INTERVENTION	NURSING EXAMPLE	CHARACTERISTICS	DESIRED OUTCOME	REQUISITE NURSING SKILLS
Health care professionals	Health Volunteers Overseas	Nurse educators holding an advanced degree work directly with nurses to advance nursing education in the host country	Improved nursing practice through collaborative education	Teaching skills Curriculum design Communication skills Capacity building Collaboration Organizational management
Voluntary organization	Small NGO*	Nurse as consultant on the board of directors	Improved service and health care to those served by the NGO	Communication skills Collaboration skills Quality and safety Management skills
Health care systems	Romania 1989 (Julia's work)	Nurse consultation with health ministry to advance professional nursing	Increase in professional nursing in country post-Communist dictatorship	Leadership skills Advocacy skills Management skills Organizational leadership

*NGO: Nongovernmental organization

Throughout the history of the nursing profession, nurses have served in a variety of roles beyond the borders of their home settings. Whether this was in other countries during war time, on the frontiers of their own countries, or in voluntary capacity across nations and practice settings, nurse volunteers have assumed, and still assume, many different roles. Each nursing role requires nursing skills, but these vary across programs. Nurses might work with individuals in direct-care roles, with communities for community-based participatory research or to intervene for population health improvements, with other professionals to increase capacity for nursing care and improve patient outcomes, or at the systems level to impact health programs. Examples of nursing roles and specific skills can be explained by the focus of the interventions (see examples in Table 3.2).

NURSE AS CLINICIAN

During the past centuries, nurses have provided direct care as volunteers; Florence Nightingale at the Crimean War is the most notable early example. This role is the most common role for international nursing volunteers. For many nurses the opportunity to serve as a volunteer using clinical nursing expertise is an effective way to begin, because it allows them to use clinical nursing skills without the need to draw upon advanced skills for leadership, consultation, and education.

Currently nurses serve as volunteers in settings both in their own countries, such as in migrant camps, barrios, prisons, and free clinics, and across borders in other countries distant to their homes. Diane Martins, PhD, RN, whom you read about in Chapter 1, spent more than 20 years as a volunteer with Traveler's Aid in Providence, Rhode Island, USA, working on its mobile medical van that provided care for the homeless in the state. Her involvement with the homeless began when she was a newly graduated nurse working in New York City and extended throughout her academic career as a nursing faculty member (Martins, personal communication, 2010). Judith Wold, PhD, RN, leads a project for Emory University nursing students and students from other collaborating universities to Moultrie, Georgia, USA, to work in migrant camps each summer (Emory, 2010). Up to 80 faculty and students provide care to many of the more than 100,000 migrant farm workers in Georgia during their 2-week health program each year. Both within-country volunteer experiences are examples of nurses using their expertise to partner with organizations or programs in need in their own states. Each example also demands that the volunteer provide ethical and culturally appropriate care. Nurses increasingly travel to other countries with health care teams to provide care at times of disaster or for those living in poverty in the developing world. Global volunteerism is on the rise, particularly during the past 20–30 years as travel opportunities have increased, as volunteer organizations have emerged in greater numbers, and as the large numbers of post–World War II nurses have reached a stage in their personal and professional lives that allows them the time and resources to travel.

According to Rhonda Martin, MPH, RN, from the Mount Auburn Hospital Travel Medicine Center in Cambridge, Massachusetts, USA, the center has seen a rise in the number of nurses seeking immunizations for travel to serve in other countries (Martin, personal communication, July 7, 2010). In the United States, the Peace Corps, founded in 1961 by

President John F. Kennedy, encouraged opportunities for Americans to travel to faraway countries to provide service to those in need. Since that time, there has been enormous growth in direct service abroad. In France, the Medecins Sans Frontieres (MSF) was developed in 1971 and has a U.S. branch called Doctors Without Borders. Carol Etherington, MS, RN, FAAN, former president of the board of directors of the U.S. program of Doctors Without Borders, is a nurse with a long history of service in many countries in times of disaster. Other international organizations, such as the International Rescue Committee, VSO (Voluntary Service Overseas), CARE, UNICEF, International Red Cross, and Catholic Relief Services, might involve nurses in planning or for direct interventions. Organizations based in the United States, such as Health Volunteers Overseas, Partners In Health, Intercultural Nursing, Inc., the Haitian Health Foundation, Partners In Development, and the Foundation For Peace, have all been created during the past 30 years and attract nurse volunteers to serve with their humanitarian programs.

Examples of volunteer settings where nurses serve as clinicians can help to explain such roles. An early example of an opportunity for nurses to volunteer in international settings was the mercy ship SS *Hope*. Begun by William Walsh, MD, in 1958, the first mercy ship called the SS *Hope* was a donated naval ship, the USS *Consolation*. It was refitted as a peacetime hospital ship from which doctors, nurses, and technologists used their skills to both teach and provide direct care. The education of local health care workers was an integral feature of the work (Project Hope, 2011). During the duration of its use from 1960 through 1974, the ship completed 11 voyages to Indonesia, Vietnam, Peru, Ecuador, Guinea, Nicaragua,

Colombia, Ceylon (Sri Lanka), Tunisia, Jamaica, and Brazil. Since 1974, Project Hope has partnered with the U.S. Navy to send volunteers globally. The organization now has a number of land-based projects and works with the U.S. Navy to bring nursing and medical volunteers onboard ships (Lukasik, 1983). Nurse colleagues have served with Project Hope for many years, both aboard the SS *Hope*, and in land-based programs.

Religious organizations, such as the Catholic Medical Mission Board, CAM International, Baptist Medical Missions International, and the American Jewish World Service, establish missions in distant lands that frequently offer health services as part of their mission. Generally referred to as mission trips or health brigades, these settings offer nurses and other health professionals an opportunity to travel short term, generally 1 to 2 weeks, to provide direct care in free-standing established clinic sites or in various community settings. Some of these require that volunteers be of a specific faith.

After they learn about a program through friends and colleagues or via the Internet, nurses can travel to the areas where that program has established projects. Programs such as Intercultural Nursing, Inc., founded in 1984 (Patsdaughter, Christensen, Kelley, Masters, & Ndiwane, 2001), offer nurses the opportunity to travel to the Dominican Republic for a 2-week stay. While in the Dominican Republic, nurses (registered nurses, nurse practitioners, and other health care providers) travel to small remote *campos* that are geographically removed from health care services to assess and treat individual patients. In programs such as this, the outcome measured is often the number of people seen in the clinics, because it is almost impossible to maintain follow-up records for the large numbers of patients seen (usually 100–200 patients daily) during a short-term intensive program. Certainly this varies greatly across programs, but long-term outcomes for patients in free care settings are most often episodic without long-term recordkeeping or easy access for follow-up. That said, the impact upon nurse volunteers and upon the people can be profound.

A particular case of the nurse-as-clinician role concerns the large numbers of nurses who respond to disasters such as the 2004 Indonesian and 2011 Japanese earthquakes that triggered devastating tsunamis; the 2005 hurricanes, Katrina and Rita, in the United States; and the 2010 earthquake in Haiti. We devote Chapter 5 to the special issues to consider for nurses who volunteer to serve in emergency settings in response to disasters.

NURSE AS EDUCATOR

Nurses serve as volunteer educators in both local and distant settings. The volunteers include not only those whose primary professional role is education, either in academic settings or in professional development, but also highly skilled clinicians who serve as clinical mentors to nurses in other countries. There are three specific educator roles:

- Educator as collaborator in health or academic settings in other countries

- International nurse faculty exchanges

- Nurse faculty-led international student experiences

Some organizations such as HVO (www.hvousa.org) have education as the foundation of their vision and mission statements (see Box 3.1). In their guiding principles they emphasize the importance of maintaining the highest practice standards, respecting other cultures, and matching the skills of the volunteer to the specific needs of the host country partners. They promote sustainable programs that build local capacity in a spirit of mutual cooperation and respect where both the volunteer and the host partner learn from one another. HVO offers nurse educators programs in two locations in Cambodia, and one each in Tanzania, Uganda, and India. Common topics requested by host partners are teaching methods, curriculum development, assessment skills, critical care skills, newborn care, home care, and specialized topics such as wounds, burns, and respiratory care. The authors each work with this organization: Julia helped to develop the nursing education program in Uganda in 2001 and currently serves as president of the board of directors, and Jeanne serves as program director for Uganda and on the HVO Nursing Education Steering Committee. In later chapters we give examples of nurses Linda Baumann, PhD, RN, FAAN, and Ellen Milan, RNC, and their work with HVO.

A second role for nurse education is that of a faculty member in a formal academic exchange. Lange and Ailinger (2001) describe a successful international exchange between faculty at Pontifical Catholic University in Chile and George Mason University College of Nursing and Health Science in the United States. They note the importance of pre-exchange planning, effective communication, academic planning, and evaluation of the exchange to build and implement effectiveness. They offer practical suggestions that include being open to building a synergistic relationship, mutual learning, flexibility, open-mindedness, identification of strengths and weaknesses, shared language, and the inclusion of social interaction beyond the academic setting. This role shares many characteristics of the consultant role, but requires specific expertise in curriculum design, innovative teaching strategies, and assessment and evaluation.

For nurse educators contemplating a sabbatical opportunity, many voluntary organizations offer long term service options that can be developed into appropriate projects. Nurse faculty can serve globally through the funded Fulbright Scholar program as well (Nicholas et al., 2009).

The final educational role is that of faculty mentor for nursing students who participate in international immersion experiences globally. This role is discussed in depth in Chapter 6. We recommend that prior to serving as a faculty mentor, the nurse should volunteer without bringing nursing students to the location. This allows faculty to assess the potential for student learning, service, and the time to create necessary partnerships.

NURSE AS CONSULTANT

Nurses are involved as consultants both at home and internationally for areas such as health service delivery and planning, strategic planning, curriculum development, infectious disease, health care interventions, disaster preparedness and response, and use of technology (Rosenkoetter, 1997; WHPA, 2007). The World Health Professions Alliance defines a consultant as "an expert qualified and experienced in a specific discipline or field to give advice or services to a person, organization, or government" (WHPA, 2007). It further defines international health consultants as experts who have specialized knowledge, experience, and personal attributes that qualify them to provide advice or services (other than direct care) beyond their home country (WHPA, 2007).

Julia has served as a nurse consultant in a number of global settings. One example of nurse consultation at a national level took place in Rwanda in early 1995. During 100 days in 1994 between April and July, more than 800,000 Rwandans were killed in civil warfare between Hutus and Tutsi factions. Following this genocide, Julia, who was serving as assistant general and chief nurse of the U.S. Public Health Service, and her assistant, Mary Pat Couig, MPH, RN, FAAN (former assistant surgeon general, former chief nurse officer, U.S. Public Health Service from the United States), were invited by the Rwandan Ministry of Health to assist them in reestablishing public health services in the country of 7 million people. At the time of the initial visit in February 1995, the government had determined that there were only eight doctors and 32 nurses remaining in the entire country. Two of these nurses had been hired by the government and assigned to collaborate with the U.S. nurses to develop a strategy to deliver much-needed public health services throughout the country. The team, comprising ministry nurses and the consultants, realized that as thorough a community/country assessment as possible was the first step to take. This included morbidities affecting the people; any resources that were available in each area such as nongovernmental organizations, both indigenous and foreign; language capabilities of the citizens and the individuals providing care; monetary resources; facilities for training; available instructors, and so on. The plan evolved over a 1-month period of time. The four nurses devised a system of providing 3 months of health education to individuals from the community. Twenty-five students were enrolled at each of five sites and received both didactic and practical experience. The course was offered in five sites throughout the country and the course was offered in each site four times during 1 year. This resulted in 500 community members with basic health training, especially in the three morbidities that comprised 94% of the illnesses that were prevalent throughout the country, as determined by the needs assessment. The prerequisite for taking the course required that the enrollee had completed secondary education, which was difficult to negotiate with the Ministry of Health officials who did not see this as a necessity. The four nurses made the point that as the country stabilized and medical and nursing schools reopened, these community health workers should be given the opportunity to advance their education in the health field. Within 2 years, a 4-year nursing program was offered in two sites in the country, and the medical school in Butare was reopened. The four nurses have remained in contact through the years and seek advice from one another as the nursing profession has grown since that consultation.

ORGANIZATIONAL COSTS

We talk in more depth in Chapter 7 about some of the logistical issues, but when you are exploring volunteer opportunities, cost considerations should be a factor. Most programs charge a set fee for volunteers that includes in-country transportation from the airport to the volunteer site and covers lodging and meals. However, this fee varies greatly among programs and is dependent upon the type of housing, the distance from the airport to volunteer location, and the logistical issues to acquire safe water and food sources.

Many volunteer organizations expect some financial support from the potential volunteer. This support might be a requirement to join the organization, and that cost can vary from less than $100 to larger costs. Many programs include a percentage of the operating costs into their participant fee, which means that participants are actually making a donation to the program with the fee to volunteer. Other organizations require potential volunteers to raise money through donations to the program before they are accepted. Still others might expect that the volunteers raise money or obtain donations of supplies.

In addition to the fee for the program, you must consider the cost of travel and airfare to the location. Some programs include travel insurance in the fee, whereas others expect the volunteers to procure their own insurance. We will say more about insurance and the importance of this expense in Chapter 7. Some programs book travel for the entire group to travel together, whereas others leave travel arrangements up to volunteers. Programs that prefer to have the volunteer team travel as a group often book the flights for the volunteers. If you have accumulated frequent flyer miles or want to vary the itinerary, these flight arrangements are an important issue to discuss with the potential volunteer program.

WHAT CAN I EXPECT IN THE PRACTICE SETTING?

You will find more information to help you better understand the practice setting for many volunteer opportunities in Chapter 8. When you investigate organizations, learn as much as possible about nursing practice expectations. While exploring the expected role, you also need to learn about the types of health issues you will encounter, the practice environment, and the other health professionals you can expect to work with. In some settings you are likely to practice in clinics or community primary care settings, whereas in other situations you might work in hospitals or other institutional locations. We talk more about this issue in Chapter 4.

HOW DOES THIS ORGANIZATION ADDRESS MY PERSONAL NEEDS?

We devote more attention to your personal needs in Chapter 7 and Chapter 8, but you need to investigate what the actual living situation will be while volunteering for any program or organization. Learn as much as you can about housing, meals, access to safe water, security, and issues such as lavatories, electricity, and telephone access. You need this information in order to match your comfort needs to what is provided by an organization. Each of us has encountered a volunteer in the field who found the living situation so challenging that it caused problems for the volunteer and for the program staff as well. This chapter has provided an overview of how to assess possible volunteer opportunities. After you have read Chapters 7 and 8, we urge you to return to this chapter to consider how to assess a positional volunteer program.

The identification of specific role expectations for nurse volunteers in volunteer settings is important to those embarking upon a new volunteer role. Knowledge of the expectations for the nurse in the host setting is essential so that you as a nurse volunteer can assess your own skill set and knowledge base and can ultimately provide effective nursing service. Once you identify the role expectations and the needs of the volunteer organization and setting, you can begin the most important phase of self-assessment for appropriate match of skills, knowledge and the needs of the volunteer setting. In Appendix B we offer some samples of international volunteer programs where nurses and other health professionals can volunteer.

BECOMING AN EFFECTIVE VOLUNTEER

- Use many sources of information such as local networks, nursing publications, nursing professional organizations, Internet resources, and published volunteer guide books to learn about volunteer opportunities.

- Examine the philosophy and history of the program or organization.

- Learn about the operational management of the program or organization.

- Identify the expected role for nurse volunteers.

- Examine the necessary expenses incurred by volunteers.

- Learn about the location, environment, and practice setting for your anticipated volunteer work.

- Examine how the organization addresses the volunteer's personal needs.

- Complete an assessment of organizational factors for each potential volunteer organization.

CHAPTER 4

MATCHING YOUR SELF-ASSESSMENT AND PROGRAM NEEDS: FINDING THE BEST FIT

In previous chapters we discussed how to assess your own motivations, physical needs, skills, and talents and the programs available to nurses who want to volunteer globally. Finding a good match between the program goals, needs, and activities and your own self-assessment is extremely important if you want to become an effective volunteer and have the safest and most rewarding volunteer experience possible. It's a good idea to refer back to the self-assessment criteria you completed in

Chapter 2 at this point. Review what you noted on each checklist to help you assess yourself as a potential volunteer. In this chapter, we suggest specific information to consider as you examine yourself in relation to the programs you are considering. We will also ask you to identify key features of each program you are considering. We will then offer a matching checklist to help you make your best choice.

Take a look back at your self-assessment. Be as realistic and honest with yourself as possible. All humans are not alike, and we each have specific talents to offer. Do not be judgmental and make assumptions about what qualities you think an effective volunteer nurse must have. For example, do not assume that an extroverted leader brings more to an assignment than an introverted good listener. In addition, some nurses love the outdoors and have camped and hiked, whereas others prefer the comforts of home and would find living in basic lodging very difficult. Most importantly, if you are reading this book and recognize that volunteering overseas is not for you, recognize that millions of other people share that view. The criteria we discuss are applicable to all volunteer settings. Additionally, not all volunteering opportunities are for everyone.

A SECOND LOOK AT YOUR SELF-ASSESSMENT

Now that you have read a bit more about nurse volunteering and completed the self-assessment and organizational reviews, it's time to filter this information in a way to match you to a program. There's no computer program to do this for you. Instead, it takes your own honesty and effort to do this effectively.

First, look again at your *motivation.* Determine which statements really reflect your motivations the best. Summarize these into a few words or phrases. We will use a fictitious nurse, Susan Morgan, to provide an illustration. Susan completed her assessment and determined that what most motivated her was her religious tradition that encouraged her to help those less fortunate. A second motivation was her desire for adventure. So she inserted the words *giving to others* and *adventure in a new country* into Table 4.1.

TABLE 4.1

SELF-ASSESSMENT: PERSONAL AND PROFESSIONAL FACTORS

SELF-ASSESSMENT FACTOR	SUSAN'S SUMMARY OF ASSESSMENT FROM CHAPTER 2
Motivation	Giving to others
	Religious faith
	Adventure in a new country
Time commitment	Family and work responsibilities
	Allow for 2-week maximum stay
Cost/ability to pay	Financially able to pay no more than $1,000 to volunteer
Personal living concerns	Not happy to live without comfortable bed, hot shower, and morning coffee
	Good physical condition; stamina, if well rested
	No chronic health issues
Social issues	Extrovert with interpersonal skills
	Nonjudgmental
	Eager to learn from people in another culture
	Likes privacy

TABLE 4.1, continued

SELF-ASSESSMENT FACTOR	SUSAN'S SUMMARY OF ASSESSMENT FROM CHAPTER 2
Personal talents	Fluency in Spanish
	Ability to engage people
	Strong ethical principles
	Spirit of adventure
Professional skills	Has been away from clinical nursing for the past 8 years while working in an administrative role
	Administrative and management skills
	Professional development
	Interpersonal skills

Practical but very important issues of the *time commitment* expected and the *cost* must be priorities before making a serious commitment to the work. Susan consulted with her family and examined their finances to determine that she could actually take 2 weeks to travel to volunteer and spend up to $1,000. She also discovered in her conversations with extended family that some were happy to help fund her trip so that her expenses would be reduced. Adding in the cost of travel medical insurance, appropriate immunizations, and the purchase of necessary supplies such as bed netting, Susan recognized that the funds she had available without her family's help might not be enough to cover all her expenses.

Despite her feelings of what she *should* be able to tolerate in a *living situation*, Susan was very honest in her self-assessment and realized that she would be very uncomfortable in difficult living arrangements such as a tent or bunkhouse, at least for her first trip to volunteer. Privacy after the work day was over was important for Susan to get needed rest to meet the challenges of the volunteer work. However, she judged herself very fit at age 50 and had no chronic health issues. She recognized that if she were well-rested she would have a great deal of stamina.

In looking at some of the *social issues* identified in the self-assessment, Susan was aware that she was an extrovert who worked with all types of people in her work setting. She had excellent organizational skills and was a skilled facilitator who could improve conflict situations. She was confident that she could fit into the volunteer team. Beyond that, she also knew that she could be a strong team builder even in her first volunteer assignment.

Susan also knew that she worked well with people from a variety of cultures in her professional role. Through the years she has learned that she indeed has sensitivity for diversity issues related to race, ethnicity, gender, and sexual orientation and that she would adapt without much difficulty to the new cultural environment. Avoiding judgmental attitudes and remaining open to new experiences were two of Susan's strongest assets. Additionally, in her work in the perioperative setting, ethical principles have been very important to her practice, particularly confidentiality and issues of informed consent. Susan rates her strong ethical principles as an asset to working with people from other cultures and those who experience disadvantages in their living or working situations or in their access to health promotion and health care.

Evaluating *professional skills* is important to estimate the contribution you can make to the volunteer team. In your self-assessment, we encouraged you to examine not only your clinical skills but also management, teaching, and interdisciplinary skills. From this self-assessment, you should now be able to summarize your professional expertise into several statements to add to Table 4.2. Though Susan moved into an administrative role, she actually was the clinical manager of preoperative services in her hospital. This information helped guide her to organizations that provide surgical services as part of their mission. In addition, she identified her attributes in management, working with other disciplines, conflict resolution, negotiation, and professional development. She added these to her matching exercise.

TABLE 4.2

ORGANIZATIONAL FACTORS

Name of program or organization	Diocese of Orlando, Florida / Surgical mission
Mission, goals, and values	The Office strives not only to empower the people of our sister diocese and improve their lives, but also to educate and encourage the members of the Diocese of Orlando to use their time, talent, and treasure to reach out to those in need.
History	Diocese of Orlando, Florida, created a sister relationship with the Diocese of San Juan de Maguana in the Dominican Republic in 1983. Since that time they have developed housing, education, and health services for those in the diocese.
Nurse role	Surgical nurse, OR team, preoperative assessment, post-operative care
Focus of nursing interventions	Direct clinical care in hospital surgical setting
Location	Dominican Republic
Expenses	$900–1,000
Personal needs	Immunizations / Housing in a hotel, some food provided, safe water source, travel from airport to site provided

IDENTIFICATION OF ORGANIZATIONAL COMPONENTS

Look back to Chapter 3 to review important program or organizational factors. There we highlighted some aspects of a program that impact your role as a volunteer. We asked you to use Table 3.1 (included here, already completed, as Table 4.2, Organizational Factors), to complete an assessment for each possible program that you are considering for volunteer work. These factors can be summarized into three broad areas: philosophy and mission, nursing role and practice, and personal factors (cost, health, safety, and travel). Making a careful study of each program helps you to find the best match for your personal goals, skills, and needs.

Returning to our example of Susan Morgan, RN, we hope to show you how to use the tools from your self-assessment and your examination of various programs to make this match. Susan explored a variety of programs that she learned about from nursing colleagues, from the Internet, and in professional nursing publications. Because she was fluent in Spanish, she decided to focus on programs in Latin America. She completed the organizational factors table (see Table 4.2) for several organizations. Offered in this chapter is her table for the Diocese of Orlando, Florida, surgical mission. Consulting its website, she learned of its philosophy and some of the program factors. The website states, "The Office strives not only to empower the people of our sister diocese and improve their lives, but also to educate and encourage the members of the Diocese of Orlando to use their time, talent, and treasure to reach out to those in need." In addition, she read that, "Participants in the Mission Office's international projects deepen their sense of commitment to God's people, both at home and abroad, and are able to respond to the call to be prophetic followers of Christ."

TABLE 4.3

SUSAN MORGAN COMPLETES HER MATCHING EXERCISE

TOPIC	PROGRAM FEATURES: DIOCESE OF ORLANDO
Motivation	Surgical missions are under the auspices of the Roman Catholic Diocese of Orlando, Florida. Location is in the western region of the Dominican Republic, about 3.5 hours from Santo Domingo. Participants need not be Catholic; however, there is spiritual sharing and reflection each morning.
Time commitment	Most trips are for 1-week duration.
Cost/ability to pay	The program fee includes the hotel, some meals, transportation from the airport in Santo Domingo to the site about 4 hours away. Total cost of the trip and flight (from the United States, and varies according to distance traveled) is approximately $900–$1,000 for 1 week, not including travel insurance or immunizations, malaria prophylaxis.
Personal living concerns	Volunteers are housed in a hotel in the town where the volunteering service takes place. Rooms are single or double occupancy, private bath, with potable water provided, air conditioned, with security provided. The hotel is a 10-minute walk from the hospital.
Social issues	Teams usually comprise 40 volunteers including about 3–6 surgeons, OR nurses and technicians, PACU nurses, surgical post-recovery nurses, and 5–6 interpreters.

SUSAN'S SELF-ASSESSMENT	DEGREE OF FIT
Giving to others Religious faith Adventure in a new country	Susan concluded that she would be comfortable with the spiritual focus of the mission group. She had never traveled to the Dominican Republic and was pleased that the program was held in a less urban area than the capital city.
Family and work responsibilities Allow for 2-week maximum stay	
Financially able to pay no more than $1,000 to volunteer	She determined that she would be able to secure the necessary expenses to volunteer with this group.
Not happy to live without comfortable bed, hot shower, and morning coffee Good physical condition; stamina, if well rested No chronic health issues	For her first trip to a poorer country, she felt that being housed in a hotel would be the best fit for her. Her concerns about safety, food, and water were also lessened after learning about the housing and safe water.
Extrovert with interpersonal skills Non-judgmental Eager to learn from people of another culture Likes privacy	The size of the team did not pose a concern to Susan because her organization and management skills help her to work with large groups effectively.

TABLE 4.3, CONTINUED

SUSAN MORGAN COMPLETES HER MATCHING EXERCISE	
TOPIC	PROGRAM FEATURES: DIOCESE OF ORLANDO
Personal talents	Language spoken in the Dominican Republic is Spanish.
	Local hospital lacks much of what nurses are used to having in more highly developed areas. This includes the lack of X-ray capability in the OR.
Professional skills	Assessment of up to 100 patients preoperatively (combined orthopedic and gynecological), surgical interventions for approximately 50 patients with postoperative follow-up, and consultation for other patients in hospital during the week.

Susan noted that the program has a Christian foundation and philosophy. Although Susan is not of the Catholic faith, she felt comfortable with what she read on the website. She learned that teams travel from various locations throughout the United States to San Juan de Maguana, Dominican Republic, to work with Dr. Alejandro Cabral Hospital there. Because the surgical teams actually perform surgical cases at the hospital, she concluded that might be a good fit for her expertise as a perioperative nurse manager. Susan contacted

SUSAN'S SELF-ASSESSMENT	DEGREE OF FIT
Fluency in Spanish	*Susan believed that her work as a manager in perioperative care would be an asset to the team.*
Ability to engage people	
Strong ethical principles	
Spirit of adventure	
Has been away from clinical nursing for the past 8 years while working in an administrative role	*Though Susan had not been involved in clinical nursing in 8 years, she considered her leadership and management skills an asset for this type of volunteer experience.*
Administrative and management skills	
Professional development	
Interpersonal skills	

the mission office to learn more. The results of her conversation allowed her to complete the table of organizational factors that you saw in Table 4.2.

Based upon this assessment and program matching exercise that we summarize in Table 4.3, Susan Morgan Completes Her Matching Exercise, Susan determined that the opportunity with the Diocese of Orlando, Florida, would be a good fit for her talents and needs. Her next step after contact with the mission office would be to complete the application, available online.

We offer the example of Susan Morgan to highlight the importance of matching your personal self-assessment for volunteer experiences to the particular needs and activities of the volunteer organization. We suggest that you follow the process we highlighted here using Susan as an example. Making an appropriate match between your skills and talents and the needs of the volunteer program is essential for ethical and responsible volunteer service. Failure to find a good fit for your talents can result in wasted time and money for both yourself and for those who need service.

BECOMING AN EFFECTIVE VOLUNTEER

- Review your self-assessment completed in Chapter 2, Thinking Seriously About Volunteering.

- Carefully and honestly consider each response as you complete Table 4.1 with your own responses.

- Review Chapter 3, Finding a Volunteer Program, to examine organizational considerations.

- Complete Table 4.2 with Organizational Factors relevant to the organization where you hope to offer your services.

- Complete your matching exercise in the same way Susan did by making evaluative summary comments in the final column, "Degree of Fit."

CHAPTER 5

NURSING RESPONSE
TO DISASTERS

–with Mary Pat Couig

Nurses have always been on the front lines serving in disaster settings. Thousands of nurses are quick to respond to a report heard on radio or television news. It might be a report that a Category 5 hurricane formed in the Gulf of Mexico is expected to make landfall in the next 24 hours on the border of Louisiana and Texas. Or, it might be the tragic news of a tsunami arriving in the Indian Ocean, reaching Indonesia and as far as India. The 12 January 2010 earthquake in Haiti and the 11 March 2011 earthquake and tsunami in the northern part of Japan captured the hearts of many people around the globe, including many nurses and other health professionals. In response to the news, you, like many others, will want to help.

In this chapter we discuss essential information that nurses must address when making the decision to volunteer or not in disaster situations and how to best be of help. Nurses serve in many roles at home and abroad in disaster response. We discuss types of disasters, general information about disaster response, essential skills for nurses to fill the required roles, preparation, actual service, and effects upon the volunteer. We speak to examples both in the United States and globally, and we offer resources (see Table 5.3) for those seeking to register for disaster relief. There are, however, many ways to offer support during times of disaster. Or you might find some services you can perform locally, and sometimes the best, most realistic option is to donate money to a reputable organization providing necessary services in the disaster area.

DISASTER DEFINITION AND CLASSIFICATION

The Oxford Dictionaries define disaster as "a sudden event, such as an accident or a natural catastrophe, that causes great damage or loss of life" (2011). In nursing we often think also of what the consequences mean for health and health services and how the event disrupts the functioning of families and communities (Veenema, 2003). Disasters can be classified into natural or man-made. Natural disasters are caused by forces of nature, and examples include floods, mud slides, hurricanes, fires, earthquakes, tsunamis, and volcanoes. As the term implies, man-made disasters are those caused by humans, but these can either be intentional or unintentional. Intentional man-made disasters include arson, deliberate release of toxic substances such as ricin or a biological agent such as smallpox, radiation exposure, and other acts of terrorism. Unintentional man-made disasters include power outages; nuclear power plant meltdowns; volatile material explosions, such as refineries or landfills; structural collapses, such as bridges, tunnels, or dams; and mechanical mass-transportation accidents, such as airplanes, subways, and trains.

Evidence indicates that natural disasters are becoming more frequent as a result of climate change, increasing population density in ecologically fragile areas, and lack of adequate infrastructure to withstand the effects of natural disasters (Greene & Greene, 2009; Robinson, 2010). Consequently, more intensive media coverage alerts us to the needs of people in all parts of the world. A disaster can result in a public health emergency, an event that threatens the lives of many and can potentially threaten national security. An infectious agent that causes a pandemic influenza is another example of a public health emergency. In the United States, the secretary of health and human services, in consultation with public health experts, has the authority to declare a public health emergency. This declaration puts into place mechanisms to respond to the event—for example, access to medical and biological products not yet approved by the Food and Drug Administration in a timely manner, such as the declaration that was issued in April 2009 in response to the recognition of a new, potentially deadly virus, H1N1(U.S. Department of Health & Human Services, 2009).

ALL-HAZARDS PREPAREDNESS

The disaster emergency management cycle includes four phases: mitigation, preparedness, response, and recovery.

- *Mitigation* is the continual process of reducing risk to lives and property. In a geographic area prone to floods, this might mean employing engineering techniques to divert potential flood paths away from homes or businesses. Everyone witnessed how the inadequate levee barriers in New Orleans exacerbated the effects of Hurricane Katrina in 2005.

- *Preparedness* is a continuous cycle of planning response strategies, training responders, and practicing response with disaster drills for potential events. Part of this process includes identifying potential hazards in your area and developing appropriate response plans.

- *Response* is the overall coordinated effort after an event happens. This involves nursing actions such as triage, direct care of patients, patient transport, and public health planning, including the provision of basic human and sanitation needs.

- *Recovery* is the process and actions taken to return the affected community to normal, and this phase includes staff debriefing, mental health follow-up, disease surveillance, and completion of evaluation plan and response.

TYPES OF NURSING ROLES AND ESSENTIAL SKILLS

Nurses can participate at any level and in any capacity of the public health emergency response system as long as they are trained and prepared. Likewise, the skill set needed depends on the deployment role. Generally, nurses provide clinical care, such as surgical, medical, maternal-child health, and mental health nursing care. Other service roles for nurses besides the clinical role include that of planner, coordinator, educator, or care manager. Nurses can also serve as members of public health assessment teams and in senior leadership positions. During Hurricane Rita, contributing author Mary Pat Couig served as the health and human services' emergency response team leader when she served as chief nurse officer for the United States Public Health Service. Registration with an organization serves as a way to match your particular professional skills with specific deployment needs. Nurses must also be able to adapt their skills in triage to settings where resources are scarce. Traits associated with nurses who are skilled at triage include good judgment, leadership, strong clinical experience, the ability to be calm under stress, decisiveness, and the knowledge of available resources (Legg, 2009; Qureshi & Veenema, 2003).

Beyond your clinical skills, you also need leadership skills, knowledge of special populations, technical knowledge, and knowledge of culture (Legg, 2009). Leadership includes the ability to be flexible, to be highly motivated, to communicate effectively, to make decisions, and to be aware of your own emotions. Knowledge of special populations such as older adults can help the volunteer to understand their special needs in a disaster, such as possible problems with mobility or cognition or the need for medications to manage chronic illness. Being open to issues of culture is also important. Though you would have little time to make extensive preparations for the culture of the population where you would serve, knowledge of general cultural considerations for all people can assist you in being open to the local culture when you arrive to help. For example, the ability to recognize that health beliefs, gender-role expectations, role of authority figures, food practices, time orientation, variation of other cultural values, and specific beliefs about birth, death, and dying provides the volunteer with the ability to be less judgmental and better able to understand cultural differences. Other nurses note skill sets that include critical thinking; knowledge of organizational design, information systems, and specific endemic diseases to the disaster area; and the ability to collaborate effectively in a multidisciplinary setting (Veenema, 2003). Rhonda Martin, who has critical care nursing skills but also has a master's degree in public health, shares her insights from her experience serving after Hurricane Katrina.

CHANGING LIVES

Rhonda Martin, MPH, RN, was one of many nurses who served as a volunteer during Hurricane Katrina in 2005. Her message is clear: Nurses who respond to disasters should be deployed with an organization with connections to the overall disaster plan and should not arrive with small groups unprepared to join into the larger emergency response. At the time of Hurricane Katrina, Rhonda was working in the ICU at a major Boston medical center. Skilled professionals from her medical center were deployed with Disaster Medical Assistant Teams (DMATs) and some with the Harvard Humanitarian Initiative. Her hospital linked her with a public health unit out of Maryland for a 2-week deployment to Gulfport, Mississippi, near the center of the hurricane damage. The assignment was to monitor public health and sanitation in the more than 200 shelters in churches, schools, and public buildings all over Mississippi.

The nursing role was to monitor infectious disease outbreaks, to assess sanitation and health risks, and to keep data for the central command. In Gulfport she wore Red Cross attire, used rented vehicles, and visited shelters throughout the state. She witnessed the hurricane disaster and found roadways littered with storm damage. As a volunteer she was housed in a church recreation hall, where the team slept on the floor and where they were provided with one meal per day in the morning. By the end of the 2 weeks, most of the hurricane survivors housed in the shelters were dispersed to more long-term housing with friends or family, and the shelters were closed. Rhonda's team was deployed to Shreveport, Louisiana, in anticipation of more evacuees from New Orleans when Hurricane Rita arrived on the Gulf Coast, but her team was sent home when there was no longer a need for its services. Her most pivotal observation was how capable the local residents were in helping their displaced residents. People living local to the shelter found ways to support the needs of the evacuees by inviting them into their homes for a hot shower or by tending to their needs. Rhonda was impressed with not only the local people and their ability to mobilize in the time of need but also how effective the organized response could be. Self-appointed volunteers who arrived in the region without connection to the broader response effort were not only ineffective but also used the limited resources (food, clean water, and other supplies) that were best used by the hurricane survivors themselves (Personal communication with Rhonda Martin, February 2011).

PREPAREDNESS

In the United States, the Department of Homeland Security has developed a *National Response Framework* that "presents

the guiding principles that enable all response partners to prepare for and provide a unified national response to disasters
and emergencies—from the smallest incident to the largest
catastrophe. The *framework* establishes a comprehensive,
national, all-hazards approach to domestic incident response"
(Department of Homeland Security, 2011). Part of this framework includes an organized system of response, the Incident
Command System. For the system to function most efficiently,
all the participants and volunteers need to be prepared and
trained before a disaster strikes. We offer information about
specific system-level disaster planning in the United States as
examples of how local, regional, and national response organizations should work together efficiently to meet the public
health emergency needs.

ARE YOU PREPARED TO VOLUNTEER?

Ideally, when you hear the announcement about the hurricane
or other disaster you are already prepared. If you have not
registered with a relief organization already, you are likely
to find that most organizations cannot use your help on very
short notice. Likewise, you should never consider volunteering
outside an organized response system (Stokowski, 2008). If
you spontaneously show up in a disaster area, the local command has to use precious time figuring out how you might be
able to help. They have to verify your licensure and determine
where to place you in the response actions. Not only are you
a drain on resources, you might not be able to use your skills
or expertise if you haven't already established yourself with a
disaster-response organization. You need to give substantial

thought to your current situation and decide upon the fit between your professional skills and the service role you wish to fulfill and your level of commitment. Your commitment can include the following issues: ability to meet any costs incurred, how much time you have to devote to getting and keeping ready to volunteer or deploy, the length of time you could be away from work and home, and the distance you are willing to travel—for example, to another part of your state, another state, or another country. You need to have personal and professional preparedness plans in place, your training needs to be up-to-date, and your gear should be packed and ready to go.

If you are not ready and prepared, you need to *honestly* assess your current family and work situation, your commitments to others, your physical and mental health, and your training and preparation. You should ask yourself how far you are willing to travel to volunteer, if you have the support of your employer for missed work, and if you have the financial resources to be away from your job (Stokowski, 2008). If you are going to help someone else in a stressful, constantly changing environment, you must be in optimal physical and mental health with minimal distractions back home. One of the cardinal rules of any volunteer assignment or deployment is not to become a burden or put yourself or others at risk. Sometimes you have no control. During Hurricane Rita, one of the deployed personnel was sent home because of a sudden severe illness in an immediate family member. Someone who is worried about a loved one back home cannot fully concentrate on the task and might endanger himself or herself and others.

To help you assess your current situation, ask yourself the questions in Table 5.1, Self-Evaluation of Disaster Volunteer

Readiness. This is not an exhaustive checklist, but it should get you thinking about your situation and how you might reasonably volunteer.

TABLE 5.1

SELF-EVALUATION OF DISASTER VOLUNTEER READINESS

Are you responsible for the care of others? Humans? Animals?

Who will be responsible while you are away?

Do you have any medical conditions that might jeopardize your health in a potentially unsafe environment?

Do you have any medical conditions that, if they significantly deteriorated, would cause you to become a casualty and consume resources and time meant for those affected by the event?

Do you have disaster responsibilities at work? Have you discussed your wish to volunteer with your employer?

How do you handle stress? How flexible are you?

Are your legal affairs in order?

Do you have liability and workers compensation coverage if you won't be covered by the organization with whom you are deploying?

UNITED STATES VOLUNTEER OPPORTUNITIES

The next step after you've made a decision about volunteering is to consider with which organization to volunteer. We highly recommend deploying on a team or as part of an organized group. Participating on a team provides the infrastructure, resources, and equipment for becoming and maintaining preparedness and provides logistical support when you deploy. Additionally, your skills and expertise can be appropriately used and professional licensure can be verified before the disaster. All disasters have potential risks. Deploying with a well-prepared and trained team can help allay or decrease those risks, both physical and emotional. Our "Changing Lives" stories throughout this chapter highlight the value of working with a team.

In addition to federal volunteer programs, such as the Community Emergency Response Team (CERT), Medical Reserve Corps (MRC), National Disaster Medical System (NDMS), Disaster Medical Response Teams (DMATs), and Emergency System for Advanced Registration of Volunteer Health Professionals (ESAR-VHP), opportunities exist with the American Red Cross or one of the many university or religious affiliated disaster-related relief organizations. In 2002, the American Nurses Association created the National Nurse Response Team that functions within the larger NDMS program (Health and Human Services, 2011). Websites for these organizations are included in the "Resources" section at the end of this chapter. A good place to start in your community is with your local public health department, your place of worship, or the chamber of commerce.

The CERT program's educational focus is on community all-hazard vulnerabilities, general incident management and command, and basic disaster response skills. Trained CERT team members can help community members before local fire and rescue responders are available to help. CERT members are encouraged to support public health emergency response agencies by actively participating in community preparedness projects. Currently 933 MRC units serve their communities. Though the focus of the MRCs is on training and preparing health professionals for public health emergencies, the units are encouraged to address other public health needs in the community, such as immunizations and blood pressure screenings. MRC members can be deployed to help during federally declared disasters.

The NDMS DMATs are highly trained community-based teams of health professionals and support staff often associated with and supported by a local health care organization. They are classified according to their capability to respond. A Level-1 DMAT can be ready to deploy within 8 hours of notification and remain self-sufficient for 72 hours with enough food, water, shelter, and medical supplies to treat about 250 patients per day. Level-2 DMATs can deploy and replace a Level-1 team using and supplementing equipment left on site. Level-3 DMATs are teams in development. Like other federal government-related assets, when members of these teams/units are deployed, they become activated as federal employees, which allows for licensure in disaster settings and coverage for liability and worker compensation.

ESAR-VHP is another federal program created to support states during public health emergencies through establishing standardized volunteer registration for licensure, credentials, accreditations, and hospital privileges verification in advance of emergency situations.

The American Red Cross is well known for disaster response and has hundreds of chapters across the country. It also offers many first aid and disaster preparedness courses.

Like other organizations, it might have training and education requirements you need to meet before you can be deployed. If you are interested in volunteering locally, you might want to consider the CERT and MRC; if you are willing to travel, you can consider the DMATs (also require a higher level of training and exercising), ESAR-VHP, and ARC. Note, however, that MRC units can be requested for deployment during a federally declared disaster.

ENSURING PERSONAL READINESS

Preparing to respond through education and training is an important component of the readiness process. We suggest that you read documents such as the "MRC Federal Deployment Competencies" (Office of Civilian Volunteer Medical Reserve Corps, 2011) and the "Disaster Preparedness White Paper for Community/Public Health Nursing Educators" (Kuntz, Frable, Qureshi, & Strong, 2008) to learn more about the specific competencies expected for nurses who volunteer in public health emergencies.

However, equally important is ensuring your legal affairs are in order. Those who have served in the uniformed services are familiar with family care plans. These plans ensure your legal affairs are documented and articulate your wishes for guardianship of any minor children or dependents for whom you are responsible. The organization you volunteer with might have a suggested format; if not, you can refer to the suggestions in the "Family Care Plan" sidebar. Whatever format you choose, make sure your legal affairs are in order before you deploy in the rare case something happens to you.

TABLE 5.2

FAMILY CARE PLAN

Make sure your will or family trust is up-to-date, including power of attorney for health decisions. If necessary, designate a guardian in the will/family trust.

If you are a guardian or caretaker (for example for an elderly parent or a special needs child/adult), make sure someone else is designated as a responsible person while you are away and make sure the guardian understands his/her responsibilities. Arrange for the guardian to have access to necessary funds.

Check to make sure all ID cards and professional licensure have not expired and will not expire while you are away.

Check your life insurance policy/policies and update beneficiaries as needed.

Arrange for housing, food, transportation, and emergency needs.

Inform your spouse or any caretakers/guardians about your financial matters.

Discuss your plans with your spouse/significant other.

PHYSICAL ISSUES

Depending upon the location and the emergency situation, you might encounter a variety of challenges in the volunteer setting. Some of these relate to the living conditions and your ability to get adequate rest. In addition, the long working hours can limit time for self and relaxation. Frequently, volunteer housing creates close living conditions and lack of privacy. Many disaster areas are in tropical climates where the heat, insects, and sun can all affect health and well-being. In Chapter 8 we address the physical adjustments and include a more extensive discussion of health and safety concerns. The welfare of the volunteer is important to volunteer organizations (Hewison, 2003), so if you as a potential volunteer have concerns about these issues, you need to discuss them at the time you register as a volunteer.

PSYCHOLOGICAL ISSUES

No matter what your clinical expertise or role in a disaster response, you will find it helpful to know about mental health issues during disasters. Both providers and those affected by the disaster might be suffering psychological distress resulting from physical injury, loss of life, safety and security, interpersonal networks, and environmental conditions in the disaster area (Plum, 2003). Victims often experience feelings of helplessness, lack of safety, horror, and stress in response to the loss of their loved ones and their homes, from witnessing death and disfigurement, and from the loss of common resources such as churches, schools, markets, and medical facilities. Exposure to these traumatic situations often affects the volunteer as well (Thormar et al., 2010). Again, relief organizations generally provide mental health support not only to those affected by the disaster but also to the disaster volunteers.

The size and scope of some disasters stretch the resources available to meet the needs. In addition, smaller organizations are likely to have fewer volunteers, and deployments might be longer and more frequent (Adams, 2007). Hopefully, the volunteer team will have a mental health provider who can attend to the needs of both those affected and those helping, or mental health resources will be available in the community.

Reactions to disasters depend on many factors including the type of disaster, the cause of the disaster, how many total lives were lost, and whether or not relatives or friends were adversely affected by the disaster. Disaster reactions can be emotional (e.g., anger, sadness, depression); physical (e.g., fatigue, worsening of chronic conditions, gastrointestinal); cognitive (e.g., nightmares, trouble making decisions, confusion); or behavioral (e.g., difficulty sleeping, substance abuse, interpersonal difficulties). Providers should be on the alert for signs and symptoms of psychological distress in both the affected population and their team members. Psychological distress in disasters is normal and in most cases amenable to treatment interventions.

PROFESSIONAL AND ETHICAL ISSUES DURING A PUBLIC HEALTH EMERGENCY

Every nurse should be knowledgeable about the American Nurses Association Scope of Standards for Practice for their clinical area and the *Code of Ethics for Nurses* (American Nurses Association, 2001). These documents provide guidance on our professional practice to help ensure the highest level of care is delivered in an ethical manner. During times of disaster, the legal and ethical obligations prescribed by these documents can conflict because of the lack of resources, overwhelming emergency demands, and the need to make difficult decisions. Under normal circumstances, patients receive the best possible care given their unique situation and the available medical products and technology. During a public health emergency or disaster, resources, both physical and human, might be limited or in some cases nonexistent. Think about pandemic influenza, the accompanying respiratory distress or failure, and a lack of ventilators. If 50 people present to an emergency department, all in respiratory distress, and that department has only 25 ventilators, how is it decided which patients get a ventilator?

At a time of limited resources, health-related decisions need to shift from doing the most for a single patient to doing the greatest good for the most individuals. The result is that some patients might not receive the optimal care they would have received under different circumstances. The Department of Health and Human Services asked the Institute of Medicine to develop recommendations regarding care delivery in a time of limited resources, and in September 2009, the Institute of Medicine released *Guidance for Establishing Crisis Standards of Care for Use in Disaster Situation* (Institute of Medicine, 2009). This document provides principles and guidance to health professionals, health care facilities, public health departments, and others on how to develop and implement policies and procedures for delivering care when resources are limited. Nurses need to understand the public health concept of the greatest good and be familiar with the general principles of crisis standards of care. A key recommendation in the report is the development of coherent state protocols based on the following: "A strong ethical grounding; integrated and ongoing community and provider engagement, education, and communication; assurances regarding legal authority and environment; clear indicators, triggers, and lines of responsibility; and evidence-based clinical processes and operations" (Institute of Medicine, 2009, p. 5).

As mentioned earlier, in the United States, the secretary of health and human services has the authority to declare a public health emergency. During a declared emergency, Medicare, Medicaid, Children's Health Insurance Program (CHIP), and

Health Insurance Portability and Accountability Act (HIPAA) requirements might be waived or modified. As part of your pre-briefing for your deployment assignment, this information should be provided; if it is not, you should ask about the current status of government health regulations and your responsibility. Depending on the type of disaster, quarantine or isolation health measures might be implemented. This happened during the H1N1 pandemic; travelers entering countries were checked for fevers and other symptoms of H1N1, and the public was encouraged to self-isolate if they demonstrated signs and symptoms of H1N1 influenza.

GLOBAL DISASTERS

Increasingly, nurses volunteer in global settings in response to disasters. As mentioned previously, we strongly recommend you volunteer with an organization if you want to volunteer to help in a disaster relief effort in another country. The International Red Cross is an organization with a long history of meeting the needs of those experiencing global disasters. In recent years, global disasters have taken many lives. The 2004 tsunami in Indonesia (300,000 deaths), the 2008 earthquake in China (70,000), the 2010 earthquake in Haiti (250,000), and the March 2011 earthquake and tsunami in Japan (more than 18,000) prompted nurses worldwide to respond to the overwhelming needs. Nurses in China responded in the first wave of rescue teams after their 2008 earthquake, playing a critical role in the relief effort (Yang, Xiao, Cheng, Zhu, & Arbon, 2010). Japanese nurses are among the more than 230 Japanese Red Cross medical teams that have responded to that disaster. One nurse who served in Indonesia with the U.S. Public Health Service (USPHS) aboard the U.S. Navy ship *Mercy* noted that not only did nurses and relief workers provide direct care to those injured in the tsunami, but also they had many opportunities to "promote the spirit of health diplomacy through our commitment to providing care to those in need...and to build relationships based upon the compassionate bedside care" (Pryor, 2005, p. 474).

When a nurse serves in an international setting, some considerations extend beyond those encountered in the home country. In addition to the issues and challenges previously described, you also need to consider language, culture, transportation, safety and protection, medical issues (immunizations and medical evacuation insurance), and country entry and exit. You can read other chapters of this book to learn more about some of these issues if you seek to volunteer beyond the borders of your home country. We offer an example of a Haitian-American nurse who traveled to Haiti weeks after the 2010 earthquake that illustrates the importance of language, culture, and traveling with an organization.

CHANGING LIVES

Stephanie Victoria is a Haitian-American nurse born and raised in the United States who works in oncology nursing at the Brigham and Women's Hospital in Boston, Massachusetts, USA. At the time of the 12 January 2010 earthquake, her hospital began to recruit nurses to go to Haiti to work with Partners In Health, an organization with a long history of service to Haiti. PIH chose to send orthopedic nurses and those who spoke Creole in their first wave of volunteers. Within days she was getting her immunizations and medications for travel and preparing her supplies, including a tent, sleeping bag, iodine tablets, protein bars, and medical supplies, and within 2 weeks Stephanie was in Haiti working at the hospital in St. Marc where many earthquake survivors were being cared for. Her experience arriving at the Port au Prince airport soon after it reopened, spending the first night in a tent in Port au Prince, and noting the chaos and upheaval everywhere, further convinced her that the only way to volunteer in a disaster was to be part of an organized team. After she traveled to St. Marc, she immediately went to work with very little orientation in the hospital, where most of the patients were orthopedic trauma patients. Though she was knowledgeable about Haitian culture and language, she was not familiar with the health system of care in terms of how the nurses cared for patients, the role of the family members as caregivers, and the pain management procedures. She tells us, "The family members are pivotal to patient care." Families are there to help with patient needs, to administer medications, and to remain with patients throughout their hospital stay.

Stephanie also notes that she had to advocate for appropriate pain management medication to get the patients moving after their orthopedic surgery, but she also had to build a trusting relationship with the patients. Because she could speak the language and knew the culture, she could better understand the patients' needs to gain their trust.

An important feature of working with the PIH team through her hospital was the debriefing process—the physical examination, and psychological follow-up offered to all returning volunteers. She notes that this process was very important to the nurse volunteers and was available because she served with an organized team.

Though her time there was exhausting and emotionally draining because of the trauma she witnessed everywhere, she found this, her first volunteer experience, very rewarding, and she hopes to return to Haiti again soon. She and other Haitian-American nurses are organizing their support for the new nursing education program to be established at the government hospital now being built by PIH in Mirabalais, Haiti.

Though it does not have political jurisdiction in global settings, the World Health Organization (WHO) has excellent disaster resources on its website as part of the Health Action in Crises and Global Alert and Response programs. The Health Action in Crises division of the WHO "works closely with Member States, international partners, and local institutions to help communities prepare for, respond to, and recover from emergencies, disasters and crises" (WHO, 2011). Their mission is saving lives and reducing suffering, working in efficient partnerships for disaster management, capacity building for countries and health systems, and advocating for political support to assure the essential resources, preparedness, management, and recovery in times of crises (WHO, 2011).

Another international resource is the Sphere Project. The Sphere Project is a collaborative effort between a number of nongovernment organizations and the Red Cross and Red Crescent Societies to define minimal requirements during disasters and humanitarian responses. Its work is built upon beliefs that people affected by disasters have the right to life with dignity and that the response should alleviate human suffering. The handbook of the Sphere Project includes minimum standards for all sectors: water, sanitation, and hygiene; food security, nutrition, and food aid; shelter, settlement, and non-food items; and health services (The Sphere Project, 2011). Reliefweb (2011) is a United Nations website that provides current information on humanitarian crises around the globe. Nurses should specifically consult the International Council of Nurses (ICN, 2011) and the International Nursing Coalition for Mass Casualty Education (INCMCE, 2011) for the specific guidelines and resources available. Please see the "Resources" section at the end of this chapter for a more extensive listing of suggested resources.

The terms *refugees* and *internally displaced persons (IDPs)* are often cited in conjunction with global disasters or public health emergencies. The United Nations High Commission on Refugees (UNHCR) is responsible for refugees, and their primary goal is "to safeguard the rights and well-being of refugees" (United Nations High Commission on Refugees, 2011a). A refugee is defined as someone who "owing to a well-founded fear of being persecuted for reasons of race, religion, nationality, membership of a particular social group or political opinion, is outside the country of his nationality, and is unable to, or owing to such fear, is unwilling to avail himself of the protection of that country" (United Nations High Commission on Refugees, 2011b). This definition was established as part of the 1951 Refugee Convention establishing the UNHCR.

When Julia was the chief nurse officer of the USPHS, she was asked to help with the Rwandan refugees, specifically the unaccompanied children, who were in the UNHCR-run camps in Goma, Zaire, after the genocide in Rwanda. Internally displaced persons (IDPs) are persons who have fled their homes but remain in their own country. Oftentimes they flee for the very same reasons as refugees. Even though UNHCR's primary focus is refugees, it has helped an estimated 14 million out of a total 26 million IDPs. Before you volunteer in another country, make sure you research the situation and the organization for the best possible outcome.

We offer reports from the recent earthquake in Haiti to show examples of concerns by nurses who volunteered their services in the weeks immediately following the disaster. Within hours and days of the earthquake, nurses were encouraged to volunteer. One agency urged people to "Make that phone call. Take that extra step, and get involved" (Herbst, 2011). Many nurses did just that and located an agency with which to serve.

A pediatric critical care nurse flew to Haiti several months after the earthquake to manage the pediatric intensive care unit in the Project Medishare tent hospital, the only functional trauma hospital in Haiti post-earthquake. Though it was effectively supplied with medical supplies and medications through its sponsorship by the University of Miami Global Institute, other materials much needed for the care of children were scarce. The medical needs were overwhelming, but this nurse noted that the enormous differences in culture and poverty were challenges for him to address to provide competent care for the children. He stated, "I was definitely not prepared for how much it was going to affect me. And I was also not prepared for how guilty I felt for being home" (Fraleigh, 2010, p. 37).

For many disaster survivors, the recovery phase can last years. In Haiti the needs remain and the need for volunteers continues. Gena Deck, RN, an ED nurse from New Hampshire, first responded to the call for nurses to serve in the immediate days after the earthquake but found that she wanted to serve long-term to help with the needs of the Haitians now living in tent cities. Learn how her first international volunteer experience in a disaster led to her continued commitment as an international volunteer in the "Changing Lives" feature.

CHANGING LIVES

Gena Deck, BSN, RN, is an emergency room nurse with certifications in pediatric and adult trauma. She was one of thousands of ED nurses who responded to the Haiti earthquake and registered through the Emergency Nurses Association to volunteer their services. She states, "I had never been on a traveling medical trip before. Prior to becoming a nurse, I was a middle school teacher of English as a second language. I have always been drawn to other cultures and opportunities to teach, and to learn. Haiti, after the earthquake, presented itself as a timely opportunity for me. I am fortunate to have a supportive family and the means to leave my job and travel to help others."

She arrived in Haiti about 1 month after the earthquake and worked for several weeks in a small clinic in Port au Prince that fortunately had survived the earthquake and was run by Partners in Development. That experience inspired her to return a few months later for a 3-month assignment, as well as 1 year later for a 2-week assignment. With her strong background in education, she saw the need to help educate and transition the new medical/nursing teams that arrived on a weekly or biweekly basis. In addition, as the clinic visits grew and more Haitian staff members were hired, she recognized that her talents could be used to help the interpreters learn about common health problems that presented in the clinic. During her 3-month stay she developed a certificate program for clinic staff members that ran for several weeks on weekends at the close of clinic operating hours. Approximately 20 Haitian staff members who worked as interpreters, lab assistants, and pharmacy assistants completed the program.

Her work shows that what began as a response to a disaster became an integral part of her professional career. Back at home she is currently completing a master's in education, focusing on women's health issues and reproductive rights/education. "I hope to teach in places like Haiti, Somalia, or other countries where there is a need, so that the students and citizens of those countries can take care of their own in the best way possible," Gina says.

Volunteering during times of public health emergencies and disasters can be extremely rewarding and challenging. Being prepared before you go ensures you are in optimal mental and physical health to give your best effort and can completely focus on helping others. Deploying with a team ensures you have the education and training to function at your highest level and ensures a support infrastructure for the team to work most efficiently. Nurses must not forget that the long-term effects of a disaster extend for years following the event. If volunteering with an emergency response team is not suited to your skills or personal life, you might consider volunteer service another time.

Additionally, you need not travel to support the rebuilding efforts. In Haiti, for example, the ICN established the Supporting Nurses and Nursing in Haiti Fund that will support the efforts of Haitian nurses to rebuild the National School of Nursing destroyed in the earthquake, and support the nursing profession to meet the needs of the Haitian people. Other ongoing programs such as Partners In Health, UNICEF, and other smaller programs such as Partners In Development and Haitian Health Foundation continue to help Haitian health professionals meet the needs of the population in Haiti. You need not travel to the site to be of help when you feel the need to respond to a need for assistance. Contributions to those organizations that continually serve on the front lines might be your best choice. Volunteering months beyond the actual event might also be the way you can help. The priority must be to ensure that the most qualified relief workers and the most organized response teams are the priority responders to disaster events.

TABLE 5.3

RESOURCES

American Nurses Association, Disaster: www.nursingworld.org/
MainMenuCategories/HealthcareandPolicyIssues/DPR.aspx

American Red Cross, Volunteer: www.redcross.org/en/volunteer

Center for International Disaster Information: www.cidi.org/about-cidi

Centers for Disease Control & Prevention, Center for Public Health Law:
www2a.cdc.gov/phlp

Centers for Disease Control & Prevention, Emergency Preparedness and
Response: www.bt.cdc.gov

Community Emergency Response Team (CERT): www.citizencorps.gov/cert

Disaster Medical Assistance Teams: www.phe.gov/Preparedness/
responders/ndms/teams/Pages/recruitment.aspx

Emergency System for Advanced Registration of Volunteer Health
Professionals: www.phe.gov/esarvhp/pages/about.aspx

International Committee of the Red Cross: www.icrc.org

Jonathan Malloch, Tennessee-1 Disaster Medical Assistance Team:
Comprehensive equipment list: www.md1dmat.org

Medical Reserve Corps: www.medicalreservecorps.gov

Relief International: www.ri.org

Reliefweb: www.reliefweb.int

United Nations, Office for the Coordination of Humanitarian Affairs:
www.unocha.org

U.S. Department of Health and Human Services, Public Health Emergency:
www.phe.gov

U.S. Department of Homeland Security, Are You Ready?:
www.fema.gov/areyouready

U.S. Department of Homeland Security, National Response Framework:
www.fema.gov/emergency/nrf/aboutNRF.htm

World Health Organization, Global Alert and Response: www.who.int/csr/
don/en

World Health Organization, Health Action in Crises: www.who.int/hac/en

BECOMING AN EFFECTIVE VOLUNTEER

- Learn about disaster classification.
- Identify essential skills for nursing in disaster settings.
- Learn about the roles nurses assume in disaster response.
- Recognize the importance of preparedness.
- Assess your readiness for volunteering in a disaster.
- Read about volunteer opportunities in the United States.
- Recognize the benefits of registering with a local emergency response team.
- Ensure your personal readiness.
- Develop a family plan.
- Identify professional and ethical issues in emergency response.
- Learn about global disasters.
- Learn from the wisdom of nurses who respond to disasters.
- Use our resources to become prepared for disaster response.

CHAPTER 6

EXPERIENTIAL LEARNING FOR FACULTY AND STUDENT NURSES

The discussion of global nurse volunteering to this point has been directed toward licensed practicing nurses. In addition to licensed nurses who volunteer globally, large numbers of nursing students participate in volunteer efforts in their own country or internationally. Many such experiences serve to engage students with communities, to offer opportunities for service, and to promote knowledge of global health.

Recommendations from nursing organizations such as the American Association of Colleges of Nursing *Essentials of Baccalaureate Education* (AACN, 2008), the American Academy of Nursing Expert Panel on Global Health (Rosenkoetter & Nardi, 2007), and the International Council of Nurses call for nurses to come together globally (ICN, 2011) to advance their knowledge and experience in global health, and in particular for nursing faculty and students to participate in greater numbers in global health volunteer efforts. In addition, the impetus from university mission and goal statements to prepare graduates as global citizens further encourages nursing faculty to provide opportunities for students to engage in global health programs. As a result of these factors, nursing programs increasingly offer opportunities for students to travel to distant areas of their own country or to other countries for formal international study experiences, for campus exchanges, and for experiential learning that can meet criteria for service learning (Seifer, 1998). In this book we focus upon nurse volunteering, but we believe that nursing students and faculty can benefit from a brief discussion of the range of experiences available to students.

In this chapter, we speak particularly to the issues that surround student experiences in global health. Though many nursing students volunteer locally or work with the underserved in their community health nursing practicum experiences, many nursing students also seek to explore other volunteer options and gain experience in more global settings.

This chapter addresses two separate audiences. First, it speaks to nursing students who have an interest in volunteering in settings distant from their home as well as those who have an interest in international health. In this chapter, we offer information to guide students to appropriate learning or service programs and briefly differentiate among global health opportunities currently available for nursing students, so that they can identify possible programs for their own learning and service. Table 6.1 outlines the various types of experiential learning and service.

Second, this chapter speaks to nursing faculty who lead student programs. Not only must faculty possess clinical expertise as teachers of future nurses, but also when hosting student experiences, they must model ethical and responsible service. Accordingly, we highlight the particular issues related to faculty/student programs in global health at home and abroad and offer guidance for practical, ethical, and responsible programming. We offer faculty some examples of U.S. university programs that model effective partnerships and discuss logistical issues that nurse faculty must consider before bringing nursing students to health settings beyond the usual university partnerships. Next, we discuss special issues related to health, safety, and appropriate supervision of students. Finally, we offer suggestions to faculty who plan to develop or revise opportunities for nursing students to improve learning for students and service for the host partners.

FOR NURSING STUDENTS

In this section, we direct our comments to nursing students who are interested in learning more about nurse volunteering, help students locate opportunities to serve as volunteers both locally and globally, offer examples of student volunteer experiences, and provide an overview of the types of programs available to nursing students.

TABLE 6.1

TYPES OF GLOBAL NURSING STUDENT EXPERIENCES

TYPE OF PROGRAM	KEY FEATURES	LOCAL COMMUNITY	WITHIN HOME COUNTRY	INTERNATIONAL LOCATIONS
Academic exchange	Often referred to as study-abroad programs, these most often include specific academic learning and course credit.			Student travels to study in another country during school semester or summer session.
Academic-sponsored clinical Practicum experiences	Most frequently these meet clinical requirements in community/public health or nurse practitioner nursing courses that place students in local or international settings as clinical practicum experience for course credit.	Often include settings with populations of older adults, children, those who are homeless, people living in shelters.	Student might participate in an alternative clinical practicum assignment in location away from home, such as with a First Nation population setting, but within home country.	Incorporated into both the school of nursing and the college or university international program office, students can meet requirements for clinical practicum in international setting.
Community service/ volunteerism	Projects that students undertake as part of their personal activities beyond the academic setting. These can also be part of community service initiatives at particular academic institutions.	Student elects to volunteer independently or with a volunteer group to provide service in local community.	Student elects to travel independently or with a volunteer group to provide service within own country.	Student elects to travel independently or with a volunteer group to provide service internationally.

TYPE OF PROGRAM	KEY FEATURES	LOCAL COMMUNITY	WITHIN HOME COUNTRY	INTERNATIONAL LOCATIONS
Experiential learning beyond academic course requirements	Experiential learning can occur in either local settings or immersion settings away from home location. Generally these are not for academic credit, such as independent study courses.	Faculty offer experiential learning opportunities for students in local community beyond specific course requirements. An example would be a faculty member who volunteers on a van to provide health services in the community and invites students for extra-curricular experience.	Faculty offer experiential learning opportunities for students in another community beyond specific course requirements. An example would be alternative spring break trips to work with Habitat for Humanity projects within home country.	Faculty offer experiential learning opportunities for students in international community beyond specific course requirements. An example would be a faculty-led international immersion experience during school break.
Service learning programs	Must meet criteria for service learning that include reciprocal relationship between academic partners and community partners, embedded in a course, uses reflection for learning, and meets community need.	Service learning partnerships in local community	Service learning partnerships in settings within home country, such as the Emory University/Moultrie Georgia experience.	Service learning partnerships in international settings, such as the program for nursing, engineering, and other students at Valparaiso University in the United States and a community in Nicaragua.

FINDING NURSING STUDENT EXPERIENCES

If you are a nursing student reading this book, we hope to encourage you to consider nurse volunteering. The rewards are great and can impact your future goals as a nursing professional. You need not leave your home or school location to become active with a volunteer organization. Faculty members at your university often can help you locate agencies or organizations where you can use your talents. In addition, if your nursing program has a chapter of the National Student Nurses Association, you can learn more about volunteer opportunities. We suggest that you read Chapter 2 to assess your interests, talents, and goals as a volunteer. Be honest in your self-assessment. You might also be interested in international health or spending time in an international setting. Everyone has different talents and interests, and you should not decide to make a trip to please your family or friends. Traveling to international settings is not for everyone. If you have any doubts about international experiences, you should probably postpone making such a trip until you are a registered nurse.

If you have carefully identified your interests and talents as you completed Chapter 2 of this book, you might find you are best suited to an educational exchange that focuses upon your own learning rather than on service. This is especially true for nursing students who have not completed at least 3 clinical courses. You can learn about international programs from the office of international programs at your university or read about some nursing examples in Appendix C. If you have completed your junior level courses and your nursing program offers an opportunity for students to travel to another location in your own country or internationally, we urge you to read more. As a senior nursing student, Jeanne spent 1 month working and living as a student volunteer with a migrant health project about 400 miles from her nursing program. This opportunity not only provided the experience of working with migrant farm workers who traveled the East Coast farm worker stream, but also helped form her lifelong commitment to the underserved and her desire to serve those living beyond the borders of the United States.

Currently, Emory University hosts a Farm Worker Family Health Program in Moultrie, Georgia, USA, for nursing students and other health professional students to work with migrant farm workers. For the past 17 years, students from Emory University, Georgia State University, Clayton State University, and the University of Georgia have spent 2 weeks in June serving the migrant agricultural workers who come to work in South Georgia. Judith Wold, PhD, RN, the director of the Farm Worker Family Health Program, notes that the program is often life-changing for students. Undergraduate and nurse practitioner graduate nursing students see as many as 2,000 people for screenings and health assessments during their stay. For many farm workers, this is their only opportunity to access health care for the entire year (read more at http://shared.web.emory.edu/emory/news/releases/2010/06/emory-nursing-students-offer-health-care-services-to-migrant-farmers-in-south-georgia.html or watch this YouTube video: http://www.youtube.com/watch?v=oVQkYAhmd3Q). This opportunity allows students an immersion experience among Spanish-speaking farm workers where they partner to promote health in this setting.

Some student nurses become involved in global health initiatives through extracurricular efforts of their school or college. Other students become involved through projects associated with their nursing courses (Warner, 2002). Donna M. Nickitas, PhD, RN, NEA-BC, CNE, Kathleen Nokes, PhD,

RN, FAAN, and Carol Roye, EdD, CPNP, RN, created an international service learning opportunity for students within the context of an undergraduate nursing course.

CHANGING LIVES

Hunter College, Hunter-Bellevue School of Nursing, a large public university located in the heart of New York City, integrates service learning into the undergraduate curriculum. During recent years, the faculty arranged for two new global initiatives involving the countries of South Africa and Haiti as service-learning projects, creating opportunities for students to partner with communities well beyond their geographic boundaries and for unique global partnerships between a U.S. School of Nursing and an international community. The school's first global partnership was with the community-based and owned Woza Moya, a nongovernmental organization (NGO) that provides care and support for people infected and affected by HIV and AIDS in the Ofafa Valley located near KwaZulu-Natal, South Africa. The project, considered a widely respected model among the network of NGOs in KwaZulu and within South Africa, provides ongoing services to orphan and vulnerable children, home-based care, HIV and AIDS information and counseling, food security, basic medicines, and paralegal and advocacy services. The Hunter-Bellevue nursing students raise money to help Woza Moya obtain the necessary supplies needed to provide direct services. Within a 15 week semester, the students raised more than $3,100 through campus bake sales, Facebook/PayPal donations, a faculty lunch, and contributions from friends and family. To raise awareness and educate the Hunter College community, the students launched a Facebook page (www.facebook.com/HunterforWozaMoya). This page served as an effective fundraising tool as well as a social network link to post relevant facts, articles, and videos on the actual project and the community of Woza Moya. Although the nursing students were *not able to physically care for the Woza Moya community, they felt connected to them nonetheless. Through effective teamwork, care, and compassion, these students learned the nursing core values of human dignity, altruism, and integrity. As they reached out by phone and e-mail to the Woza Moya founder, Sue Hedden, and their partner organizations, Ubuntu Charlotte, with Catherine Anderson, and with the South Coast Foundation director, Kathy Cook, the students came to recognize how nonprofit agencies are managed and supported. Despite not having their feet on the ground in South Africa, the students came to understand, appreciate, and support the mission of the Woza Moya Project. Suddenly, their fundraising activities, education and awareness campaign, and social networking had removed the geographic boundaries. The global partnership between the School of Nursing and Woza Moya resulted in a meaningful service-learning experience for the students and huge financial outcomes of the project—global service-learning experience without ever having to pack a bag, travel, and leave the ground!*

Their second global service-learning project began in the fall of 2010 as a result of the devastating earthquake in Haiti. With the collapse of the main nursing school at the Hospital del l'Universite d'état, the students were moved to respond with a global relief effort all their own. When they learned that what remained of the school was without electricity and plumbing, had no Internet service, and had very limited school equipment and supplies, they raised money to help rebuild the nursing school from more than 250 fans on Facebook and through the design and launch of a website called "Promoting Health in Haiti." The student champion for the project—a student who has family in Haiti—stated, "With the right motivation, at the right time, and for the right reasons, all things are possible. We can achieve amazing things even in the shortest amount of time."

Donna notes that, "I am completely humbled and overwhelmed by the success our students have in leveraging their team-building skills to organize and implement outstanding service-learning projects. They begin their global service-learning experience oriented to core nursing values with a true appreciation of social justice. As their faculty member, I am most proud of how our students care and contribute to the relief of the world's poverty. Global nursing can and is happening in American schools. Our students can support nurses, nursing education, and public health with their heads, hearts, and hands right here at home. There is no need to travel to make a difference. We have!" (Donna Nickitas, personal communication, 2011)

Although this learning lacks the direct immersion into a new setting, with increasingly innovative media technology, students can be linked to more remote settings. Most importantly, it helps students learn the value of partnership with the people in their own home communities who are most able to make sustainable change for themselves. For those considering an international experience, an upcoming sidebar about Mary Vrana should help you recognize the impact immersion service programs can have.

CHANGING LIVES

Mary Vrana, BSN, RN, of the United States is a good example of a nurse whose experience as a senior student has shaped her nursing career. Mary first volunteered in the Dominican Republic in 2005 as a senior nursing student at the University of Massachusetts Dartmouth (UMD) College of Nursing. As a child she visited Jamaica with her family and was very concerned that children were bathing in dirty water at the side of the road while she was being served meals at a resort setting. This incongruity led her to seek an opportunity to volunteer in a poorer country.

She joined Jeanne, a faculty member from UMD, and six other nursing students, three other faculty, and other nurses for a 2-week service immersion trip. This experience involved travel to a rural area of the Dominican Republic with the group, Intercultural Nursing, Inc. (INI). Her experience as a volunteer learning about the culture and health and illness in a rural tropical setting launched her long-term commitment to volunteer service. Ever since her first student trip, Mary has returned to volunteer as an RN to the same location each January with INI. She selected her full-time employment based upon her desire to make one or two service trips each year. In addition to her yearly trips to the Dominican Republic, she has been to Haiti twice with a UMD volunteer group and with the organization Partners In Development on a total of nine volunteer trips to Hispaniola.

Mary is motivated by her love of the people she has met through her travels. She wants to better understand the relationship of culture and health, and she enjoys learning to work with what is available locally and helping empower the people she works with in the host country. Her nursing expertise, genuine love of the people she serves, and infectious energy make her an asset to any volunteer team. She looks at health holistically and solicits all sorts of donations including hats, sunglasses, socks, and shoes as ways to improve health and well-being for those served. As an avid soccer player, she brings soccer balls for the children and loves to join in the action when the day's volunteer efforts have been completed. Now she has recruited her brother to work with local construction efforts and her aunt, who is a physical therapist, to join the team in service there as well. She tells everyone that her student experience changed the course of her nursing career (Mary Vrana, personal communication, 2011).

We recommend that nursing students seeking an international experience speak with nursing faculty members within their own nursing programs. If your school does not offer a student experience such as Mary's, you might learn of a program that is open to you. We urge you to read the section directed at faculty and also students in appendixes C and D to identify whether a volunteer experience is right for you. If you are able to locate an opportunity, we recommend that you read this entire book to learn as much as possible about nurse volunteer preparation and service.

BRIEF OVERVIEW OF PROGRAMS AVAILABLE TO NURSING STUDENTS

Nursing students can participate in international programs in a variety of ways. Not all include volunteer service, but there are opportunities to volunteer as well as learn about global health issues in many experiences. This section will help you learn about university-sponsored programs, opportunities where you may be able to earn academic credit, and university and international exchange partnerships.

UNIVERSITY-SPONSORED INTERNATIONAL PROGRAMS

Most undergraduate nursing programs do not offer the flexibility for nursing students to participate in semester-abroad programs. Those seeking this type of program often find intersession and summer offerings in international settings. University-sponsored international or global health programs provide an excellent resource for students looking for such actual exchange programs, but most focus upon academic learning and do not include a service component. For nursing students, these programs are often scheduled for summer breaks so as to not interfere with required academic courses during the regular semesters.

ACADEMIC CREDIT

International student experiences sponsored by nursing faculty in college settings often provide students an opportunity for academic credit. Schools such as the University of Wisconsin (2011) offer global health courses through the Center for Global Health. Other schools such as the University of Pennsylvania (2011) offer stand-alone courses that include some form of in-country or international experience. Still other programs provide students an international option for their community/public health clinical practicum experience. Offering academic credit increases the need for faculty to prepare for costs and liability and to define goals and objectives for the program. We give examples of this type of program later in this chapter.

ACADEMIC PROGRAM TO COUNTRY EXCHANGE PARTNERSHIPS

Schools such as Villanova and Valparaiso have developed partnerships between their own university and universities in other countries. Individual students or faculty-student groups can travel to the partner country to expand their global health knowledge and experience through an ongoing formal partnership. The Villanova partnership in Nicaragua, featured in the sidebar coming up, pairs nursing students with engineering students for a project that involves a safe water initiative and cell phones for *promotores* (community health workers*)*.

CHANGING LIVES
Villanova University Nicaragua Teamwork

Villanova University offers nursing students various international learning options during their academic career. One example of a nursing student international learning opportunity is based in Nicaragua and is led by Elizabeth Keech, Bette Mariani, and Ruth McDermott-Levy. The Villanova nursing and engineering students have teamed together to serve the health needs of the local population in a variety of ways. In 2002, the Villanova engineering students began a service-learning experience in Waslala, Nicaragua. The local population identified access to clean drinking water as its most urgent need. For the past 8 years, mechanical engineers have designed and installed gravity drainage water distribution networks to improve water quality and access.

Nursing students joined the project to address health promotion concerns for the people of remote villages in the surrounding region. As part of their community health clinical course (or practicum), nursing students developed course materials and taught local community health workers (CHWs) safety, first aid, environmental health, disaster preparedness, and infectious and water-borne disease prevention and management. In a recent project, student nurses have partnered with business and engineering students to develop a method of transmitting health information from remote villages to a licensed health professional using cell phone SMS texting. The student nurses have been working with the CHWs on this telehealth project. They have taught the CHWs basic health assessment so they can transmit accurate findings. CHWs work in settings distant to hospitals and licensed professionals and are often faced with urgent health problems in their communities. Using cell phone text messaging allows CHWs better access to important professional support.

Student nurses assess the learning needs of CHWs and their understanding of health issues in the area. Using qualitative methods, Ruth and a nursing student determined the information that the CHWs believe is essential for them to access appropriate support from medical professionals. "Professionally, it has been very rewarding to meet the needs of the CHWs while working closely with faculty and students from nursing, engineering, and business on this project," said Ruth. Elizabeth, along with two other nursing students, has created basic forms for CHW documentation and is developing a method of measuring health outcomes to determine the effectiveness of the program. These specific projects have resulted in independent studies for three credits for the three students. Collaborating with nursing faculty, two of the students have presented their work at a national conference for the American Public Health Association.

This example highlights the importance of meeting the expressed needs of community members first with the issue of access to clean water, and next with the stated needs of the CHWs. Building the partnership between the university students and the Waslala community has led to better programs for students and improvements that are likely to aid health. Presently, nursing faculty members are developing outcome measures to document the positive effects of health promotion efforts, of the clean water project, and of the telehealth project for CHWs. Linking health and sanitation efforts builds sustainability for improved health (Elizabeth Keech & Ruth McDermott-Levy, personal communication, January 2011).

The following websites provide more information on this program:

- *www.villanova.edu/engineering/service/waslala.htm*
- *www.villanova.edu/nursing/newsevents/news. htm?page=2010_12_6.htm*
- *www.villanova.edu/nursing/newsevents/news. htm?page=2010_03_20.htm*
- *villanovanursing.blogspot.com/2010/06/essential-first-steps-to-improve-rural.html*

Valparaiso University also has a partnership between university students and various communities in Nicaragua. Teams that include engineering, business and health professional students are able to offer more comprehensive service to community partners. The upcoming sidebar on Valparaiso should help you learn about how sustainable projects can emerge from such partnerships.

Valparaiso University Nicaragua Teamwork

Valparaiso University's (VU) nursing program partners with the VU engineering students on their wind energy and stove projects. Mechanical engineering students who work with the group Engineers Without Borders have worked in a remote area of Nicaragua to meet the needs of the local people there. Working with a regional coordinator for International Service Learning, the engineering students developed the project that resulted in the construction of a solar-powered wind turbine monitoring system and the installation of three wind turbines for electricity in the community. The nursing and premedical students joined the engineering students in service to the same Nicaraguan community. The health professional students worked with licensed medical personnel to assess and treat health problems in the region during past years of the service trips. Building upon the culture of the community, nursing students have used poetry and sociodrama for public health education as well. "By working toward the health goals of the community, we have been able to build a project that will not only be sustainable but beneficial to the community. Developing a partnership with the community has helped us truly see health-related issues through the eyes of its people in their environment," said Tricia Erdmann, a graduate of the nursing program. In addition, under the leadership of Amy Cory, PhD, RN, CPNP-BC, PCNS-BC, assistant professor of nursing, the nursing students have developed a community-based participatory action research project in partnership with the community leaders in the local Nicaraguan village to address their leading health issues (Amy Cory, personal communication, 2011). Read more at www.valpo.edu/news/news.php?releaseId=4231

FACULTY/STUDENT EXPERIENTIAL LEARNING

Many of you reading this book might have years of experience with student nurse experiential learning in settings both in your home country with diverse populations or internationally. Others might be in the program development process. Accordingly, we offer useful information both to those with extensive experience and to those in the planning stages. We make recommendations based upon the collective wisdom of our faculty colleagues who participate in experiential learning.

INFORMATION FOR FACULTY

Nurse faculty members share student international experiences at nursing conferences and also publish descriptions and outcomes of these programs (Ailinger & Carty, 1996; Haloburdo & Thompson, 1998; Riner & Becklenberg, 2001; Bosworth, et al., 2006; Wright, Zerbe & Kornewicz, 2001). We find that the range of student immersion experiences include those that offer academic credit and those that do not; those that meet requirements for a community health nursing clinical practicum and those that do not; those that are offered outside of the formal curriculum but with university collaboration; and those that meet service-learning criteria. Though some faculty members report international student learning experiences in the literature, hundreds of others exist without any dissemination beyond their school, program, university, or the Sigma Theta Tau International website. We found it difficult to locate any central reporting mechanism for these individual programs that would be helpful to guide faculty who develop such programs. Additionally, the goals and objectives, student activities, and outcome measures are not always available beyond their local program and vary widely.

During the 2007–09 Sigma Theta Tau International (STTI) Biennial, Jeanne served with nurses around the world on the International Service Learning Task Force that produced an executive summary for the STTI board of directors to help reach consensus on international service learning for nursing. (See Appendix D for an important discussion about the criteria for service learning.) Hallmarks of service learning foster better outcomes for both student learning and for host partners (McKinnon & Fealy, 2011). Additionally, in our comments to students we offer descriptions of various program types that can help nurse faculty who are in the planning process to determine what best meets their program needs.

REASONS FOR EXPERIENTIAL LEARNING IN INTERNATIONAL SETTINGS

Why leave home? We have heard many critics suggest that nursing students need not travel internationally to engage in service learning or to work with disadvantaged communities. Though it is true that most community health nursing practicum experiences foster engagement with communities, immersion experiences come with particular benefits. One argument for service that occurs away from home is that students face fewer distractions when immersed in an experience away from their home setting. These distractions of their everyday life include access to the comforts of home, instant contact with friends and family through cell phones and social media, and the ability to freely move into and out of the host community. Such distractions can diminish the significant impact experienced in an immersion situation. For students, living within and experiencing a new culture and living environment simultaneously increase the impact of the experience and the opportunity to truly learn about another culture.

Casey and Murphy (2008) report a number of benefits of service learning for nursing students. These include an increased appreciation of civic responsibility, cultural awareness, self-confidence, interpersonal skills, and critical thinking. In many cases nursing students report their desire to return to the location of their service or to pursue future international study or work (Riner & Becklenberg, 2001; Callister & Hobbins-Garbett, 2000).

Though literature reports student benefits for service learning that include increased knowledge of community health needs, respect for diversity, understanding of personal biases, and enhanced critical thinking skills (Sigma Theta Tau International Service Learning Task Force, 2009; Nokes,

Nickitas, Keida, & Neville, 2005; Peterson & Schaffer, 1999), fewer authors report benefits for communities (Hamner, Wilder, & Byrd, 2007). However, Narsavage, Lindell, Chen, Savrin, and Duffy (2002) report results from graduate student service-learning projects that demonstrate positive outcomes for the community to meet unmet needs.

RECOMMENDATIONS FOR FACULTY AND STUDENTS

Faculty members who coordinate service-learning partnerships for students need to consider a variety of issues in order to provide students with safe, effective, and appropriate learning and service opportunities. If faculty members wish for the learning experience to be one of service learning, they must aim to ensure that the criteria for service learning (see Appendix D) are met in the educational experience. We offer specific recommendations beyond the actual educational criteria to help those who plan international immersion experiences. These recommendations include the importance of meeting institutional requirements, ethical concerns, identification and reduction of risks, safety, emotional well-being, culturally appropriate behavior, and returning home.

INSTITUTIONAL REQUIREMENTS

Whenever nursing faculty create or participate in experiential learning opportunities for students for credit or noncredit experiences, school and university requirements must be met. For matriculated students throughout their academic career, including school breaks, the institution bears some liability for student safety and well-being. Sponsoring faculty must ensure that the international programs office at the student's school or college is a partner in the experiential learning program. Students often benefit by having school-sponsored health insurance, travel insurance, and opportunities to prepare for their health needs and by learning about international travel through the university office.

In addition, if students earn academic credit for their experiential learning, they might need various forms and approvals prior to the experience. As noted previously in this chapter, some schools or colleges of nursing offer a particular course in an international setting. Others provide an option for students to use their experiential learning as their community/public health nursing clinical experience. (See the following Georgetown University program in Nicaragua sidebar.) Though credit is awarded during the semester when the student enrolls in the community/public health nursing didactic course, it might be necessary for the clinical practicum experiential learning to occur during a school break for scheduling reasons. Finally, some faculty members create independent study or topics courses that include preparation, immersion learning, and follow-up to meet specific course outcomes.

CHANGING LIVES
Georgetown University in Nicaragua: Partnership Between Nursing Programs in the United States and Nicaragua.

Rita Ailinger, PhD, RN, first served as a nurse volunteer in Nicaragua in 1966 aboard the SS Hope. She admits she was not even sure where the country was located and did not speak any Spanish prior to her interview as a potential volunteer. Once she was assigned, she quickly learned all she could, and she became fluent in Spanish through her work in Nicaragua and other countries in Latin America.

Fast forward to 1995, when Rita was a nursing faculty member at George Mason University (GMU) in Fairfax, Virginia, USA, and you will see that her expertise working in Nicaragua made her a perfect mentor for a Nicaraguan graduate nursing student, Lidya Zamora. Lidya spoke to Rita about creating a GMU nursing experience in Nicaragua in collaboration with the Universidad de Politecnica de Nicaragua. At the invitation of the vice rector of the Nicaraguan university, Rita and fellow faculty member Suzanne Molloy, PhD, RN, led student groups for 12 years to Nicaragua each January for 2 weeks. The partnership moved from George Mason University to Georgetown University when Rita became a professor there in 2007. The 2-week experience met the requirements for a community health clinical practicum at GMU; at Georgetown it provides more than 40 hours of clinical experience and many cultural experiences. U.S. students are required to be moderately fluent in Spanish, as no translators are used.

In Nicaragua, students worked in an impoverished squatter settlement (barrio) where people live in shacks, have potable water only a few hours a day, and have multiple health problems due to poverty and malnourishment. Nicaragua is the second poorest country in the Americas after Haiti. The community leaders welcome the students each year, and students work closely with the community health promoters (brigadistas).

In the barrio, each student was assigned a family with whom the student worked every day in a home visit. The student performed health assessments on family members and referred them for lab exams, prevention programs, and treatment, and did extensive health education.

In addition to visiting families, students worked in the local public health center each day, rotating through the various clinics, including epidemiology, where persons with TB and STI are seen; the oral rehydration clinic, where children with diarrhea receive hydration; and women's health, including prenatal, postpartum, family planning, and vaccination clinic. In each of these clinics, students give appropriate care and learn about the local system of health care. They also visit a local tertiary care public hospital for women and a private hospital to learn about hospital conditions.

Each student gives a health education presentation, in Spanish, at the health center and at a health fair in the barrio's nursing center. Students prepare their presentations on topics based on local health needs. A health fair was planned by a group of recent students with the help of the local health promoters (brigadistas), and 60-150 people attended.

To prepare for the 2-week immersion clinical experience, the nursing students participated in pre-trip seminars, prepared a health education project, and learned about the history and culture of Nicaragua. The first seminar focused on general preparation, objectives and assignments, completion of university documents, and a visit to the travel clinic. The second seminar was directed toward learning about the Nicaraguan culture. Each student became the "expert" in one area, such as history, the arts, literature, music, politics, and culture. They presented their findings at the pre-trip seminar and then served as the expert while in Nicaragua.

In addition, graduate nurse practitioner students worked as consultants for the undergraduate students, worked with local nurses to collaborate about both acute and community nursing care, and worked as advanced practice nurses.

This is an impressive model where U.S. and Nicaraguan nursing faculty work collaboratively as equal partners to provide culturally appropriate nursing care and education to those they serve. This program offers opportunities for U.S. students to learn from the Nicaraguan nurses as well as to provide service to others. It is a life-changing experience in social justice for many students, leading to careers in public health and working with vulnerable populations. While faculty receive stipends for their work and students gain academic credit, this work qualifies as global volunteering, as both faculty and students share their time and talents during their semester break.

Read more about this project in the following publications:

Ailinger, R. L. (2002). U.S. nursing students in Nicaragua: A community health clinical experience. Rev. Latino-Am Enfernagem, 10(10), 104-105.

Ailinger, R. L., & Carty, R. M. (1996). Teaching community health nursing in Nicaragua. Nursing & Health Care: Perspectives on Community, 17(5), 236-241.

Ailinger, R. L., Gonzalez, R., & Zamora, L. (2007). Health and illness concepts among lower income Nicaraguan women. Qualitative Health Research, 17(3), 382-385.

Ailinger, R. L., Molloy, S., Zamora, L., & Benavides, C. (2000). Nurse practitioner students in Nicaragua. Clinical Excellence for Nurse Practitioners 4(4), 240-244.

Ailinger, R. L., Molloy, S., Zamora, L., & Benavides, C. (2004). Herbal remedies in a Nicaraguan Barrio. Journal of Transcultural Nursing, 15(4), 278-282.

Kollar, S. J., & Ailinger, R. L. (2002). International clinical experiences: Long-term impact on students. Nurse Educator, 27(1), 28-31.

Nursing faculty who seek to create such experiences for nursing students should work with the international programs office at their particular school or college to begin their planning. Equally important is to learn from other programs. We offer examples of three programs from Villanova, Valparaiso, and Georgetown universities (see previous sidebars in this chapter) that we believe are excellent models for faculty/student programs. Appendix C provides various Internet resources that identify global programs at universities around the United States. In addition, we recommend that interested or experienced faculty consult the references to gain wisdom in the development or improvement of faculty-led student learning programs. In particular, we urge faculty and students to learn more about service learning and how to integrate the principles of service learning to build stronger partnerships for student learning and to meet community needs.

ETHICS

We believe that the ethical concerns that underpin program partnerships for licensed nurses apply to all student experiences as well. Factors we consider essential for ethical practice experiences are as follows:

- Those served control the services rendered by the volunteers.

- All aims for the program are transparent.

- Those who provide service must have the appropriate credentials to perform the service.

- Those who serve are learners as well as providers.

We emphasize these factors throughout this book and offer additional suggestions in Chapter 7 and Chapter 8. Crigger, Brannigan, and Baird (2006) emphasize that nurses must broaden views of nursing to blend Western health care with the culture and people who are their global partners, rather than have "commercialized Western health care transplanted into other cultures" (p. 15). Ethical concerns increase for faculty-student programs. Faculty members are not only serving as individual volunteers but also as role models, mentors, and supervisors for students. We believe that modeling ethical and responsible service for students participating in global learning programs cannot be overemphasized. We must emphasize that we are guests in the host community, have an openness to other health modalities, use appropriate technology, and respect the culture of our partners.

Nursing faculty members who support learning programs for students often face a moral dilemma when meeting the dual aims of student learning outcomes and responsible service to their host partners (A. Mason, personal communication, 2010). Jeanne has been involved with nursing student international service programs for many years. As the faculty mentor for students, she is concerned with their learning, their safety, and their well-being. Simultaneously, she must make the concerns of those served an equal priority. Though this is similar to any faculty clinical role where faculty members supervise students who deliver nursing care to patients, the issue of being a guest in another setting or country increases the challenge of meeting the needs of students and host setting members. We recommend that faculty work to achieve cultural competency skills and are able to communicate at an intermediate level in the language of the host country (Calvillo et al., 2009). We recommend that faculty who supervise student trips have at least 3–5 years of relevant experience and also make a trip to the host location prior to assuming the responsibility of leading student immersion experiences. Alicia Curtin's story in the sidebar below illustrates the importance of building partnerships, a hallmark feature of service learning that improves student learning as well as meets community needs.

CHANGING LIVES

Alicia Curtin, PhD, GNP, is an example of a nurse who has worked for 20 years to build relationships with community members in a remote area of the Dominican Republic near the Haiti border. This important example of relationship building is essential for nurse volunteers, particularly for student nurses, to experience. Alicia had an interest in serving in the Peace Corps but was unable to commit to a long-term assignment at the time, so she sought a short-term opportunity to serve in an international setting. Having studied Spanish in school, she preferred to volunteer in a Spanish-speaking country. She first visited the area in 1991 as a graduate student in nursing with the group Intercultural Nursing, Inc. (INI) to learn more about cultural issues in health, to advance her fluency in Spanish, and to identify ways that nurses could contribute to improving health in the community there. During the past 20 years, she has built relationships in the community. This experience has been most important to an elective opportunity for nursing students in this specific community in the Dominican Republic.

For the first 10 years that Alicia volunteered with INI, the collaboration between the visiting teams (those who made trips to the community each fall, winter, and summer) and the community members was essential to the work. Nurses and nurse practitioners traveled to campos (small villages) in distant regions of the parish community to host clinics in schools and community centers. Representatives from the town community joined the nurses and worked with the promotore in the campos. Though Alicia volunteered in the campos, she worked in the town as well to build relationships with the local people.

In 1994, she spent 1 month working in the local hospital to learn about the health issues common in the community and to work with the local nurses. This led to the establishment of friendships with many nurses and community members as well as the prenatal clinic, breastfeeding support, and immunization clinic staff at the hospital. In 2001, nursing students from the University of Rhode Island, Fitchburg State University, and the University of Massachusetts Dartmouth joined the nurses and nurse practitioners in the work. Alicia facilitated opportunities for students to work with the nursing staff at the prenatal, the breastfeeding support, and the immunization programs. During the past 10 years that students have joined the team, she built relationships with a Missionaries of Charity nutrition program where malnourished children live residentially, with a preschool program that has grown into an early education program through elementary school, and a program for adult day care. Students learn about the needs of the community through their work in these partnered experiences. Though the student nurses also travel to the campos and assist the RNs in their assessments of client needs, they are able to learn the importance of relationship building and meeting community needs through these relationships.

Alicia recognizes that it takes a great deal of time, a deep respect for the fact that the community best knows its needs, and a desire to let community members lead the development of the relationship in order to build relationships with global partners. Her goal is to build a stronger partnership between the university and community agencies, to increase opportunities for community members to share their expertise with students, and to potentially develop a joint community-based action research project in the community (Alicia Curtin, personal communication, 2010).

RISKS

The issue of risks to health and safety are a serious concern for any nurse traveling to a location beyond home. We discuss these issues in depth in Chapter 7 and Chapter 8. We urge you to read those chapters for a more comprehensive discussion of the topic. In this chapter we speak to some of the health and safety risks that can be more problematic when younger nurses and students are participants in international projects. Other authors report these concerns as well (Casey & Murphy, 2008). Though all of the safety factors are also concerns for licensed nurses who elect to travel as global volunteers, they significantly increase the responsibility for faculty who lead student trips. Preparation for the unexpected greatly reduces the potential for problems encountered during the global experience.

SAFETY

Safety is a concern for students in any practice environment, whether they are in their own home setting or one far from home. As part of the preparation for all clinical practicum experiences, students learn to prepare for personal safety and that of the clients they care for to promote health and well-being. Entering a new setting increases the risks to personal safety because of differences in cultural expectations, the role of men and women in other settings, transportation, and types of crime. In Chapters 7 and 8, we discuss safety issues in depth. However, for faculty who lead groups of students to distant locations, particularly across national borders, we want to address some particular situations.

Through our years of experience with global volunteering, we have learned from nursing colleagues about situations more likely to occur when traveling with students. These include personal relationships with men or women, safety alone or at night during unscheduled time, and transportation concerns. For example, in poorer countries road traffic accidents are a leading cause of injury or death. The steady increase in the use of small motorcycles or mopeds that offer little protection to the rider, the lack of a helmet-use policy, and the increasing traffic congestion in lower income countries result in serious disability and death to citizens. Students should never be allowed to ride on these vehicles.

In addition, in many countries students travel in vehicles without seat belts, often standing in the back of an open truck over mountainous roads. In many cases, ensuring personal safety when travelling is impossible, but these travel safety issues should be considered nonetheless. Students must be prepared for the need to be very vigilant about their safety, even while just walking on sidewalks. In many village communities, sidewalks might be in seriously dangerous condition, and we have witnessed holes as large as 4 feet in diameter and 4 feet deep that can cause serious injury to those not vigilant. In addition, in our travels we have both experienced motor vehicles veering onto sidewalks to dodge traffic on the road.

HEALTH—FOOD, WATER, AND TROPICAL DISEASES

When planning a faculty-led student experience, faculty must make comprehensive plans to protect the health of the students and to prepare them for the likelihood of infectious disease. This certainly includes the endemic conditions such as malaria, typhoid, or other diseases that volunteers prepare for by becoming immunized or taking prophylactic medication. Beyond those tropical or endemic conditions are risks for diarrheal or respiratory illness because of unsafe food or water, the change in dietary intake, and the living conditions at the volunteer site. As we discuss in Chapters 7 and 8, preparation must include plans for illness while on assignment and having access to appropriate treatment. When faculty members are the responsible parties while away at the volunteer site, they must be well prepared for injury and illness among both the students and themselves. We provide in-depth information about health and safety concerns in both Chapters 7 and 8 and recommend that students and their family members thoroughly read these sections.

EMOTIONAL WELL-BEING

The commonly used term *culture shock* (Heuer & Bengiamin, 2001) describes that emotional reaction that a visitor might experience when arriving in a new setting. Many nurses have described becoming upset because the standards of cleanliness, sanitation, and housing vary greatly around the globe where people live in overwhelming poverty. For many students, a trip to a poorer country for learning, to provide service, or for service learning might be the first trip away from home. Many students need several days to adjust to their surroundings and must have supportive faculty with whom to share their concerns. Many students share these feelings freely with faculty members, but many others do not share them for fear that they are not meeting expectations. Jeanne is always prepared for such concerns and schedules short meetings soon after arrival in the new setting, where she speaks about uncomfortable feelings that students might experience and encourages them to share their concerns with her or other members of the team. Regular opportunities for reflection and sharing are essential for not only students but also all participants in volunteer settings. We also require students to keep private journals for reflection and to help them process their feelings. We devote more discussion to culture shock in Chapter 8.

In addition, the unexpected often occurs. For some students, it is their first experience seeing death. When a child brought to a clinic or in a hospital setting dies, it can cause overwhelming feelings of grief and sadness. Jeanne has had experiences in the Dominican Republic and in Haiti where nurses and nursing students were working in primary care clinic settings to help with health assessment, education, and management of health problems, rather than with emergencies; however, because the clinic contained the only health professionals nearby, people with serious injuries arrived by mule, motorcycle, or in someone's arms. Such a situation might be the first time a student nurse observes a serious emergency or death. In January 2010, those in other parts of the world were reminded that disaster could strike unexpectedly when the earthquake in Port au Prince, Haiti, occurred. Jeanne was about 50 miles away in the Dominican Republic, where she felt the earthquake, but no damage occurred, and the nine nursing students were all safe. However, at that same time both students and faculty from Lynn University in Boca Raton, Florida, serving in Haiti were killed by the destruction of the earthquake (CBS News, 2011). As faculty members we must have plans in place for emergencies, for student safety, and for emergency communication with student families and the university.

CULTURALLY APPROPRIATE BEHAVIOR (ATTIRE, CONVERSATIONS, AND ALCOHOL)

We discuss the importance of culturally appropriate dress and behavior in more detail in Chapters 7 and 8, but issues related to hosting student experiences raise these and other concerns. Faculty members must take leadership in preparing students for cultural norms for dress in the host setting. In some cultures women must keep their hair, legs, arms, or shoulders covered; wear skirts or dresses; or wear long pants, but not shorts or tank tops. Men often need to be made aware of appropriate attire as well. During recreational time in a host environment, you also need to ensure that tee shirts do not have offensive designs or wording, shoes are safe for the environment, and attire is appropriate for the culture.

In some volunteer settings, students might have opportunities to interact socially with the local residents where they are living during their program. Though this interaction can be a rewarding opportunity to learn about the people and culture, faculty need to take precautions to ensure culturally appropriate student behavior surrounding the use of alcohol, tobacco products, or other substances. In addition, students should be required to consider how their language can promote or hinder what nurse experts call *cultural bridging* (Leffers & Mitchell, 2011). Communicating and posting photos on social network sites such as Facebook can cause culture misunderstandings. Increasingly, international partners become friends on Facebook, and you need to be respectful of culture when posting comments or photos. We offer more discussion of this very important issue in Chapter 8.

Through many years of experience with student groups and consultation with other faculty members who are involved with student programs, we have learned about many unexpected situations, problems, or issues. Faculty must anticipate and prepare for the possibility of potentially negative situations. For example, although students might be required to travel with a group when walking in the local town or area, students have been known to walk alone, to visit with other young men or women from the community, or to go to local places to visit, dine, or dance and then leave with a local person rather than anyone in their group. Additionally, with a generous spirit, students have given money to local people, shared their personal contact information in their home country, or in other ways possibly endangered themselves or the group as a whole.

Finally, students must be guided in learning what personal information is appropriate to share in other cultures. Topics such as politics, religious views, romantic partner information, or sexual orientation might not be mutually understood across cultural perspectives.

DIFFICULT REENTRY

In Chapter 9 we discuss many aspects of reentry into one's own home culture, particularly if the immersion experience involved service in a poorer community or location where community members lacked basic shelter, food, water, and sanitation resources. Nursing students who return from their first immersion experience in a developing country often face a period of up to several months where they are integrating their immersion experience into their lives. Faculty leaders who have shared the same immersion experience must be available for follow-up meetings to assist the students as they transition home again. For many student participants, the lessons learned stay with them and foster respect for other cultures, increase their understanding of consumption and waste, and launch lives of service to others in both small and larger ways. Occasionally, but not frequently, an immersion experience might reinforce negative stereotypes of the population that the volunteer program served. Obviously, this is not the desired outcome, and we believe that adequate preparation can reduce the chance that this might happen. In particular, the more students learn about the history and culture of the people with whom they work, the more likely they are to learn respect for and cooperation with those served.

QUALITY, ETHICS, AND RESPONSIBLE PROGRAMS

For readers who represent nursing faculty, we offer the following questions to help guide you to creating or improving programs for students. The checklist in Table 6.2 offers reminders of issues we have discussed in this chapter and will discuss further in future chapters. Your response to this checklist and efforts to achieve the highest score possible can raise standards for all nursing student global service and learning. The highest possible score is 75. Obviously, if particular criteria are not items you elect to include in your program, then the highest possible score would be lower; you can adapt our checklist to meet your own goals and needs. We offer this checklist as a guide for your own assessment of student programs and assume you will identify the best goal(s) for your program.

Despite the often challenging logistical details for planning and implementation and the specific risks for those involved, experiential learning for nursing students in global health settings can be a significantly educational, personally rewarding, and life-changing experience. Former student participants have even obtained degrees such as an MPH in international health and a PhD in nursing with an international focus and have continued to participate in international nursing service.

TABLE 6.2

EFFECTIVE, ETHICAL, AND RESPONSIBLE SERVICE FOR NURSING STUDENTS (0 = LOWEST, 5 = HIGHEST RATING)

QUALITY CRITERIA	0	1	2	3	4	5
What is the strength of the partnership between the academic institution and the host partners?						
Do we have outcome indicators for the host partners and for student outcomes?						
To what degree do we prepare students for the historical and political issues of the host partners?						
To what degree do we prepare students for the cultural factors of the host partners?						
How strong is the sustainability for this program?						
Have we met all academic institutional requirements for health, safety, and liability?						
Do students earn academic credit for their work?						
What is the percentage of students who participate in the global service program?						
Do we have ways to engage students who do not directly participate in the program while remaining in the home country?						
Do we have scholarships available for student travel?						

QUALITY CRITERIA	0	1	2	3	4	5
Do we engage the university community in the project?						
Have we created a handbook for students who participate?						
What is the extent of planning and regulations to promote health and safety?						
How well do we prepare students for the emotional impact of the experience?						
Do we have post-experience debriefing and follow-up support?						

BECOMING AN EFFECTIVE VOLUNTEER

- Learn about a variety of global health student experiences.
- Read more about service learning.
- Locate volunteer opportunities.
- Recognize important concerns for faculty mentors.
- Plan for student learning, institutional requirements, and safety.
- Learn from our "Changing Lives" examples.
- Read more in our appendices.

CHAPTER 7

PREPARATION AND LOGISTICS

–with Rhonda Martin

For those nurses who volunteer locally, much of the practical information about travel and packing that we share in this chapter is not necessary information. Despite this fact, we believe that the information about culture, health, and safety is relevant to any volunteer assignment. We urge all nurse volunteers to read this chapter. For those planning to volunteer somewhere away from home, we help you move from your selection of a potential volunteer assignment to your actual travel and departure. Though specific organizations and programs offer their own preparation guides and planning meetings, we offer our insights from years of service that includes more than a dozen countries. In addition, our nurse colleagues around the globe have added some of their suggestions as well.

Successful volunteer experiences follow careful and extensive planning for health and safety, for efficient travel, and for learning about the culture of the volunteer setting. Though we provide extensive discussion of all aspects of your planning process, we urge you to consult the resources provided by the organization you are volunteering with and also to speak to experienced nurses who have worked with the organization. The more you learn ahead of time, the less affected you will be by unexpected situations, allowing you to be more effective in your service.

MOVING FORWARD WITH THE DETAILS OF YOUR VOLUNTEER ASSIGNMENT

As you begin to make arrangements for a volunteer placement, you will encounter several necessary forms, procedures, and actions you must complete in order to move forward to your actual assignment. Some of these details are time-sensitive and also time-consuming. For prospective volunteers, the planning process frequently can take up to 1 year prior to the assignment. In this section we discuss the application process, expenses, and how to manage the costs and issues of licensure and professional practice abroad. We also discuss donations to the volunteer project that support the work of the organization or go directly to the people being served.

MAKING APPLICATION

After you have determined the best program to match your needs and your skills, you need to move ahead with the formal application for the program. This process can be time-consuming for many organizations and should be completed months before your anticipated start date. All organizations have someone with whom you can discuss your plans. Be clear on what your expectations are and what the organization expects of you. Many organizations have extensive application procedures and schedule volunteers many months or years ahead of anticipated service.

Health Volunteers Overseas (HVO), for example, has a Washington, DC, staff that receives your application with your request for the particular program. Then the U.S. program coordinator contacts you. For example, Julia was the past coordinator, and Jeanne is currently the Uganda contact person in the United States. For applicants wishing to volunteer for the Uganda program, Jeanne will call the potential candidate to respond to any questions he or she might have and will also make a final assessment of the candidate's qualifications for participation. This process can take a month or more depending upon the steps of the process. Next, the HVO office staff communicates with the Uganda volunteer country coordinator to determine the time and nursing need situation in Uganda. Issues such as the number of volunteers from the United States and other countries working at the hospital and university at any given time, space availability for housing, and in-country transportation all contribute to the precise timing for the volunteer assignment. After the official acceptance and dates are determined, then the volunteer can proceed with scheduling flights, securing housing, and making at-home arrangements.

Medecins Sans Frontieres (MSF), Doctors Without Borders in the United States, also has a structured application process. After the candidate meets the general requirements and the specific professional requirements, MSF conducts information sessions for candidates, provides an online application, and then completes a screening of candidates. After a person passes the screening process, he or she undergoes an applicant interview. After a candidate is accepted, MSF holds a briefing, and the candidate is placed in a volunteer pool until a match is found between that candidate and the need in the field.

So, we highly encourage nurses to begin the application process early. It is your responsibility to negotiate the terms of your assignment with the organization and, if possible, with the site where you plan to volunteer. Your time and expertise are valuable, and you want them to be used appropriately. In the example of HVO, the in-depth discussion with the program coordinator, the use of the online resources, and the negotiation of all details prior to the assignment make the actual experience more effective.

For those nurses who volunteer in response to disaster, the time for extensive preparation is short between application and departure. For those of you who are considering service in disaster response, we urge you to read this chapter to learn more about preparation overall, to register immediately with a relief organization, and to make general preparations for possible service. Chapter 5 addresses issues specific to volunteering in times of disaster.

MANAGING THE COSTS: FINANCING, SCHOLARSHIPS, AND DONATIONS

The next thing to consider after you have applied for a particular volunteer program and negotiated the terms of the assignment is the cost that you will incur for that volunteer assignment. Some programs offer a stipend to the volunteer based upon the length of time in service. Medecins Sans Frontieres offers a stipend, and volunteers must commit to a period of up to 12 months to receive that stipend. VSO

International, another aid organization, offers a stipend depending upon the assignment location and time involved. Other organizations might offer scholarship money for particular services. Another source of funding might be your home institution, such as a college or hospital corporation. Some volunteers have spoken to local service organizations, such as their local Rotary International or Lions Clubs International, to seek sponsorship funding and then return to speak with organization members about the work once they return home. Other volunteers contact their family, friends, and church community to assist with the costs of travel and the needed donations for the actual volunteer experience. Many have been successful in seeking sponsorship of their trip from these sources.

Raising money for your trip also raises awareness in your community of the need for experienced professionals to volunteer their time and expertise in places that have asked for help. If you strongly believe in the mission of the organization that you will work with, consider fundraising to be part of your service to their goals. For many nurse volunteers, their community, church, hospital, or university sponsorships have led to partnerships between their home community and the service organization. These partnerships strengthen the human and financial support for the volunteer organization and its mission to serve.

DONATIONS

Donations of monetary and nonmonetary items are almost always appreciated and often very helpful to the overall success of your volunteer experience. However, the decision to bring donations not specifically solicited by your organizational partners can also have some unintended negative consequences. The University of Wisconsin Global Health program offers guidelines for donations as part of its "Towards Best Practices in the Center for Global Health" (available at http://centerforglobalhealth.wisc.edu/186.htm). The guidelines note that "While these donations are procured with benevolent intentions, unexpected downstream effects, complications, and difficulties may accompany such donations" (Center for Global Health, 2009, para. 2). Various pitfalls include material donations, medical equipment and supplies, and pharmaceuticals. Problems associated with material donations include the ethical dilemmas altering the therapeutic relationship when gifts are given to patients, strangers, and colleagues. Also, material donations or gifts can set up unrealistic expectations for future volunteers. Donated medical supplies pose future costs to the host partners, such as equipment that requires extensive technical expertise and maintenance, costs for supplies for single-use products such as laboratory reagents and glucometer test strips, and items that are inappropriate to the setting. Donations of pharmaceuticals can be particularly dangerous. We discuss this in other chapters as well, but medications brought into a host setting may be labeled in a language not understood by those using them, may lack adequate refrigeration or clean water for use, may be commonly used by volunteers but uncommon in host settings, or end up in unregulated markets rather than with the intended recipient. The Center for Global Health (2009) offers five core principles for all donations, adapted from the World Health Organization's guidelines of 1999, that state that all donations should

1. Be of maximum benefit to the recipient

2. Respect the wishes and authority of the recipient

3. Not create double standards in quality or sustainability

4. Result from effective communication between donor and recipient

5. Not create future expectations that cannot be met

In recognition of the fact that donations can have unintended consequences, we emphasize that many donations meet these guidelines and can greatly contribute to sustainable growth of the organization's goals. We urge you to communicate with your volunteer organization to learn more about its need for donations and its policies before you elect to bring them along.

In the section on packing later in the chapter, we suggest that you travel light, but we also urge you to bring the requested and appropriate donations if you can. We suggest that you bring the maximum that weight restrictions allow. Some airlines extend the weight limit somewhat for medical supplies and donations if you make arrangements ahead of time. We urge you to think of sustainable donations. For people working in tropical countries, items such as sunglasses, caps to shield the sun, cotton socks, or reusable tote bags can be very helpful. Additionally, nurse volunteers have enlisted friends, church members, or other people at home to make hats and other layette items for newborns. Michelle Belletete, RN, who has volunteered for many years in Haiti, enlisted women in her church to assemble sewing kits that included fabric, matching thread, zippers, needles, and other essentials, so that Haitian women could design and make their own dresses or skirts. Additionally, the churchwomen made tote bags out of sturdy fabric to withstand heavy loads. Donations such as these empower the women in Haiti to do for themselves rather than simply receiving a donation. Michelle's work is featured in an upcoming sidebar.

CHANGING LIVES

Michelle Belletete, BSN, is an example of a nurse whose first step into volunteering became a career. Michelle was inspired to serve in global settings when she was moved to tears while on vacation in Hong Kong many years ago, as she watched small (boat people) children carry babies on their backs while begging for money. Her reaction was not only profound sadness but also the conviction that she needed to help in some way. She could not realize that dream until about 20 years later, when she learned of a short-term opportunity in Haiti.

Traveling with Intercultural Nursing, Inc., and a small group of nurses, she began a commitment of more than 20 years to the people of Haiti. During those years she made more than 30 trips, often twice a year or for long-term stays, to serve with the nuns at the children's home and Jude Anne Hospital in Delmas, Port au Prince, and in other settings. In addition, Michelle has accepted long-term assignments with Doctors Without Borders in the Democratic Republic of Congo, Zimbabwe, and Haiti as well. Her most recent work was in Haiti from April to June 2010, when she volunteered in post-earthquake recovery. Throughout the years, she has cared for thousands of people who have had joyful events, such as births, and those who could not survive serious problems, such as burns, malnutrition, and other injuries. Michelle tells potential volunteers that it is being, rather than doing, that is important and that the relationships with people matter most.

Her stories are many and range from her long-term friendship with one of the nuns she worked with in Haiti and whom she has visited in South America over the years, to that of a child she cared for over the span of more than 8 years who, as she was dying, awaited Michelle's return to Haiti to be there with her in her final hours. Michelle's service to INI as president for 3 years and her long-term commitment to Haiti have inspired many other volunteers and engaged her church congregation to provide donations and to create a legacy for nurse volunteers (Personal communication, February, 2011).

In some cases the donations are medications, medical supplies, and equipment that are useful for the duration of the actual trip but also for the long-term needs of the host partner site. Cash donations can be used to purchase medications and supplies in the country; that method is preferable, as medications and supplies purchased in the country are in the primary language and are familiar to the local population. Additionally, this money then supports the local economy.

Most organizations require that donations be appropriate to the country and locality needs. Nurse colleagues in poorer settings often creatively develop materials when supplies such as tubing, cannulas, masks, and gloves are not available. In many situations, however, donations of much-needed supplies are very important. HVO sends nurses to work with the Special Care Babies Unit nursing staff in Uganda. Some of the volunteers have been able to solicit essential medical supplies for acutely ill newborns. Oftentimes, donations of educational materials are highly valued. Jeanne was able to send enough stethoscopes and sphygmomanometers to supply the new nursing skills lab at Makerere University Department of Nursing. Noting that they lacked a model for pediatric assessment, she brought a dark-skinned baby model along for the students to learn physical assessment skills. Additionally, providing the

Haitian clinic staff at the Partners In Development clinic in Port au Prince with a Kreyol version of *Where There Is No Doctor* (Werner, Thuman, & Maxwell, 2010) provided the interpreters the opportunity to learn in their own language about many common conditions.

NURSING LICENSE

If you volunteer outside of your own state in the United States, you must be sure that you have a nursing license that is valid for your work. Further, if you volunteer in a disaster setting, you need to verify that you are licensed to practice. If you volunteer abroad, many countries require that nurse volunteers to their country acquire a local nursing license and register with the nursing council or licensing authority in that country. This procedure can take some time. You need to start the process as soon as you know that you are going to a particular country. The organization where you plan to volunteer should assist you in obtaining the necessary license to practice. Taking this important step of submitting the paperwork in a timely manner demonstrates a respect for the profession and for the people of the host country. Other locations might not require a nursing license in the country where you serve, but the organization will most certainly require a copy of your license to keep on file. The organization in turn communicates officially with the local ministry of health or health agency for the country, where they secure permission for visiting health professionals to practice.

Additionally, the International Council of Nurses in Geneva, Switzerland, has more than 130 member countries, representing more than 13 million nurses worldwide. All of these countries have a nursing association. Take the time to contact the ICN to learn something about the association in the country where you plan to volunteer. The staff can provide you the name, address, and current officers of the association. The ICN website, revised and updated, provides nursing knowledge, news, and resources in an accessible format. The council aids nurses in making global connections to nurses in other countries. Robinson (2010) notes that nurses around the world have increased their participation in global health collaboration. The Royal College of Nursing recently published a guide for nurses, midwives, and other health professionals for humanitarian work in response to this trend (RCN, 2010).

We have been very impressed with the work of the Uganda National Association of Nurses and Midwives (UNANM). The UNANM was established in 1964 and became a member of the ICN in 1969 (Zuyderduin, Obuni, and McQuide, 2010). Its mission is to "improve the welfare of nurses and midwives, to promote the code of ethics for health professionals, and to enhance quality health care by uniting nurses and midwives across the country to share experiences and ideas" (Zuyderduin et al., 2010, p. 420). The Ugandan nurses and midwives who volunteer their time to work for their professional association are indeed serving the health needs of the Ugandan people. You might find it a great help to you to make contact socially with your professional colleagues. We agree that our most effective service in international settings occurred when we collaborated with nurses who work in-country. Our international partners are the experts about their needs and how we can best be of help.

BECOMING AN EFFECTIVE VOLUNTEER

After the details related to your assignment are in place, you must prepare effectively for your volunteer service. Advance preparation is a critical component if you want to be an effective volunteer. Familiarize yourself with the history and the culture of the country. The U.S. Department of State website has country profiles for most countries. They provide a wealth of information about the population, the history, the language, and especially the culture, as well as statistical data that will be very helpful to you in your assignment.

PROFESSIONAL PREPARATION

In Chapter 1 we speak of the importance of learning about the common health problems in the location where you are planning to volunteer. Learning about tropical illnesses and their management is essential for effective nursing practice. As we noted in Chapter 1, Claire Bertschinger directs the Diploma in Tropical Nursing certificate program at the London School of Hygiene and Tropical Medicine. For those nurses living near London, participating in the course can be a real resource.

CHANGING LIVES

I was certainly geared to treating patients as I had been taught, from a "Western developed country with rich resources" perspective. I was not prepared for the most appropriate treatments for local emergencies or the secondary treatments when the local remedies failed. Early on in my service term, the experienced team left for the outside clinic in a remote area of the coast. I was left to staff the hospital. Not long after they left,

I saw a group of people quickly carrying a hammock up the road. With little language to help me, I waited in anticipation until the screaming and wailing elderly man in the hammock was laid on the emergency bench. They were all wailing and screaming. All were trying to tell me what was wrong. The gentleman's leg was badly swollen, and there was a very large black ulcer almost the length of his shin. Armed with my dictionary, I eventually found that a stingray had stung the man, and I didn't know what to do about it. There were no books or other resources to tell me what to do. The agitation continued with cries for me to do something. Help!

Haltingly, I eventually uncovered the facts behind the injury (it had happened 10 days prior and had been treated with ground coffee rubbed on the wound). I did all I could do—hospitalize him, clean the wound, and treat it with a broad-spectrum antibiotic—and the doctor was pleased with my actions when he returned. After a few days of cleaning the wound and regular antibiotics, the wound healed well and the patient went home—on foot. After this, I was hungry to learn how to handle as many different possible scenarios as I could to help me in similar situations in the future. It was then my thirst for learning commenced. I was keen to learn anything and everything and to teach my colleagues all that I knew. I often thought I would have benefited from a programme of learning before I embarked on such a tour of office in such a remote bush village, but learning on the spot benefited me well, and we eventually started a small nursing school for the local assistants so that they could manage a range of situations themselves (Elizabeth Rosser, personal communication, 2010).

Conversely, a nurse volunteer who lacks knowledge of the types of health problems that might be encountered can feel isolated and saddened. Petra Frankhuizen of the Netherlands writes of her recent experience with the cholera epidemic in Haiti, and of a nurse who felt unprepared for her assignment.

CHANGING LIVES

Today I am in Haiti. It is stressful work here. People have gone through so many difficulties. First the earthquake, now the cholera outbreak. The team I am working with works hours around the clock. Then a newcomer arrives. It is her first mission. I can see she had difficulties adjusting. She has to play a role she is not used to. As a nurse, she is supervising the national nursing staff in a cholera treatment center. All of the national staff members have more experience with cholera than she has. She tries to change the way the nurses work. "Not so many IVs! Please write a handover report!" Good ideas, but the nurses are so busy and tired of the white faces coming in, changing things. At night I hear her cry. We are so busy with our own tasks; we didn't have eyes for her difficulties. Even though we live all together, it is still very possible to feel alone (Petra Frankhuizen, personal communication, 2011).

In each of these cases, the patients were not harmed, but the outcome could be tragic if the nurse volunteer lacks sufficient knowledge and is faced with a situation where no medical personnel are available to consult. For those nurses who volunteer in remote settings, the classic book *Where There Is No Doctor* (Werner, Thuman, & Maxwell, 2010), in print since 1992, can be helpful. This manual, used by health workers and clinicians worldwide, offers information and graphics for many tropical conditions not seen in more developed, colder-climate countries. That said, volunteers should always seek to learn as much as possible about conditions such as cholera, malaria, parasitic infestations, and other health problems likely to occur in the tropical volunteer setting.

In addition to learning about endemic conditions in the volunteer setting, you need to prepare for the professional role you are going to assume. If you are to provide direct care, you must consider any necessary reference materials you might need. Learn as much as you can from former volunteers about what is going to be expected of you. Bringing along your own stethoscope and sphygmomanometer or other assessment supplies is important. If you are teaching, you might need to bring along textbooks that you can consult and then donate upon departure. Additionally, loading a flash drive with teaching materials, slides, resources, and guidelines is helpful in your teaching role. Consider bringing a second flash drive to make copies of all materials and leave it with your host partners. Even in the poorest countries and remote locations, computer technology is becoming more available, creating opportunities for the sharing of knowledge and resources electronically.

CULTURAL PREPARATION

The most important preparation involves learning about the people in the place where you plan to volunteer. This includes reading about the culture, learning about the history and political issues of the location, and studying the common health problems likely to occur there. The most important advice we can offer is for you to recognize that you are guests of the people that you serve and that they are likely to teach you more than you teach them. Though nurses from wealthier countries often have access to greater technology and the latest scientific evidence for practice, the host country nurses are experts in the health concerns of their patients. Learning to work as partners is the most effective way to improve health. We highly recommend the book *The Spirit Catches You and You Fall Down* by Anne Fadiman (1997). The book fairly depicts two perspectives of illness and helps the reader to identify how culture impacts health and illness.

Increasingly, the nursing literature includes information on culture to improve the care of patients whose culture differs from that of the nurse. This is not limited to ethnic differences. Culture also includes gender, sexual orientation, physical and cognitive ability, and lifestyle differences. Recall from Chapter 1 the example of Diane Martins, PhD, RN, who has worked with people who are homeless. Though the people she serves might only be living a short distance from her home, they experience a culture and life far different from her own. She recommends that nurses who come to work in this setting read accounts such as *Rachel and Her Children* by Jonathan Kozol (2006), *Tell Them Who I Am* by Elliott Liebow (1993), *The Mole People: Life in the Tunnels Beneath New York* by Jennifer Toth (1993), or *Down and Out in America: The Origins of Homelessness* by Peter Rossi (1991) to better understand the people and culture of living without a permanent address.

Appendix A lists a number of references that discuss aspects of diversity such as cultural awareness, cultural sensitivity, cultural humility, and cultural competence. We believe that respect for diversity begins with a desire to learn about other people and their lives. Openness to other perspectives is crucial to understanding that your own approach might not be the only effective one and that you can learn from others. Second, we believe that identifying strengths first, rather than weaknesses, helps build relationships and common solutions.

We urge you to read as much as you can about the location and people where you plan to volunteer. This is the most important aspect of preparation!

Myriam Jeannis, a senior nursing student who came to the United States from Gonaives, Haiti, in 2003, has also volunteered in Port au Prince, Gonaives, and Guatemala during the past 4 years. Completing high school in the United States, she went on to study nursing. During her college years she not only volunteered in Guatemala and Haiti, but also began a service project for young girls to attend school back in her home community in Haiti. As a Haitian woman and an American nursing student, she has a unique perspective that most nurse volunteers lack. She states, "We all have our comfort zone, and we are not likely to feel at ease when we move beyond it. Volunteering is all about this, though, leaving your comfort zone. Though you might feel overwhelmed emotionally and physically by the challenges you face in a new setting, find ways to move beyond your own needs and focus on the people you are there to help" (Myriam Jeannis, personal communication, 2011). We speak again about the effects of culture in Chapter 8, but preparation can help you adjust to a new culture and better understand the effects of what is often called culture shock.

CHANGING LIVES

Here are Myriam's tips for those who want to travel to another country to volunteer:

- *Try to learn simple words of the language the people speak.*

- *Try to understand your own cultural beliefs to identify ethnocentrism.*

- Try to leave all ethnocentric feelings behind.

- Find a local group of people who are from the country where you are interested in doing your volunteer work. Interact with them. Try to learn the most you can about their culture before you travel to their country. Reading a book is fine, but it will not provide you with all the do's and don'ts of the country.

- Complaining or whining about issues in the host country or culture is very impolite, because you will be able to return home in 1 or 2 weeks, but this is their home forever. When you belittle their home with your attitude, it is offensive and leaves lasting hurt.

- Be aware of your body language and your dress code, because it can be offending to the others' culture.

- It is OK to feel emotional and angry. However, it is inappropriate to show these feelings in front of the people you are helping.

- Avoid culture conflict.

Myriam further encourages nurses to think upstream, an analogy she uses to note that a large number of health problems should be addressed "upstream" to where the root causes occur (McKinley, 1994). She believes that the advantage of this concept is that your contribution is long lasting and valued by the community. Health promotion plays a huge role in the upstream thinking. When you go in a community to help, it is essential to observe if the symptoms you are trying to alleviate or the disease you are trying to treat is common in the community.

"Traveling to Haiti and Guatemala for the past 4 years to volunteer in clinics as a nursing student helped me to understand *that giving out ibuprofen and acetaminophen does not solve the problem of the people, because that only addresses an immediate need. Instead, if you do teaching sessions on common diseases and help them to find natural remedies to alleviate symptoms or self-manage diseases, you are making lasting changes for future generations. The reason is because when you help people to understand their body and how to take care of it, you are helping them to create a connection with their inner self and to gain a sense of control over their lives. You enable them to make decisions that change their life and their families' lives forever.*

The reward of health promotion is that you do not have to be the one to care for the person's illness, because you know the contribution that you made is endless. It can progress from one community to another. Remember, you are not there to change the entire country, but if you can make a difference in the life of one family or a community, you are their hero" (Myriam Jeannis, personal communication, 2011).

Beyond a nonjudgmental and positive approach to learning from the host country partners, we urge you to learn as much as you can specifically about the country, as Myriam suggests. Nurses who volunteered in Haiti after the January 2010 earthquake witnessed a very different Haiti from the proud country that gained its independence in 1804, which had strong sugar cane and coffee industries and hosted tourists to its beautiful land and coastline. Centuries of political strife, dictatorship, and unrest were all precursors to the devastation from the earthquake and contribute to the current situation. Without knowledge of the political and economic forces of change that affect a country, it is easy to misjudge the current circumstances of people's lives. Consider preparing yourself to understand the country and the culture in three specific ways.

1. First, locate books or articles about the location where you will volunteer. Try to learn about some of the important customs, religious beliefs, and celebrations in the host country.

2. Identify significant historical, political, and economic factors that led to the development of the current economy.

3. Most importantly, as Myriam suggests, try to meet people in your home country who have come from the country where you will serve. Talk with them and try to learn the history of the people you will serve in your volunteer assignment.

LANGUAGE

In addition to learning about the history and culture of the location where you are volunteering, you need to be able to communicate on a basic level with those you are going to work with. If the language spoken differs from your own, we recommend that you learn at least 50–100 common words in the host country language. You need to be able to greet people, ask basic questions, and respond to common questions. Bring along a dictionary to help you understand the language of your host partners. Your efforts to engage in basic conversation show your hosts that you want to work *with* them, rather than to come in from your home country with a plan to do *for* them.

Talk to as many people as possible before you go, especially former volunteers to that country. They can provide you with insight into the programs, goals, and responsibilities that they experienced and much more. The staff of the organization that you select should be able to answer any questions you have about the assignment. Remember to remain neutral on political and policy matters when you are on assignment.

PLANNING FOR YOUR HEALTH NEEDS

Attending to your own good health while on assignment is imperative. You can carry out your tasks only if you are healthy. If you have any chronic conditions or physical disabilities, you need to assess very carefully whether you can handle being in an environment without special accommodations. For example, you might be required to climb several flights of stairs when no elevator is available or the elevator is out of order. Sidewalks and roads might be in bad repair. In Kampala, Uganda, where some of the nurses who offer advice have served as volunteers, it is common to walk as many as 4 miles daily to and from volunteer sites to do marketing and to gather supplies. The terrain is often bumpy, and the city is full of hills. Further, your accommodations might require you to climb onto bunks or crawl into tents. If these are areas of concern to you, discuss it very carefully with the sponsoring organization.

One of the first topics on your to-do list should be a visit to a travel medicine clinic. Each volunteer participant should plan a personal visit so that individual needs can be met. Even savvy travelers benefit from updated vaccination recommendations, prescriptions, reports on outbreaks, country-specific regulations, and changes in the distribution of disease.

Those new to traveling and living in the developing world can expect advice on topics such as recommended immunizations, food and water safety, insect precautions, self-treatment for traveler's diarrhea and dental emergencies, malaria prevention, post-exposure prophylaxis and safe sex, personal medical kits, medical evacuation insurance, safety and legal issues, hazards of air travel, and culture shock.

The following sections include information and advice intended to assist a global nurse volunteer participant with planning and preparation and is by no means intended as a substitute for a travel medicine clinic visit, individual personal preparation, and the advice given by the sending volunteer program. The topics discussed are comprehensive, but not exhaustive. Plan to bring enough of any prescription medications to last the entire time of the assignment and some extra in case of any delays in returning home. Also, it is a good idea to bring over-the-counter medications you commonly use such as aspirin, acetaminophen, antihistamine, and topical ointments. They might not be readily available at many of the sites.

IMMUNIZATIONS

Most patients presenting to a travel medicine clinic are usually just concerned about getting vaccinated. This is normally the first topic covered by the travel health specialist before proceeding on to other important preventive and safety measure topics. Immunizations are categorized into three areas: routine, recommended, and required. Routine immunizations include common childhood vaccinations usually received at the pediatrician's office. If you were not exposed to certain childhood diseases or if you were not vaccinated against them, you are at risk of contracting the illness, especially if you travel. Routine vaccinations include measles, German measles, mumps, chicken pox, tetanus, diphtheria, and pertussis (whooping cough).

Recommended vaccinations include polio, typhoid, hepatitis A and B, meningococcal, Japanese encephalitis, rabies, and pneumococcal. Seasonal influenza and H1N1 are still a worldwide concern, and vaccination is recommended pretravel. Air travelers should be aware that close quarters and commonly used facilities increase the possibility of coming in contact with viruses. Bring a mask and sanitary wipes in the event you are seated near another passenger with respiratory symptoms.

Required vaccinations include those necessary for legal entry into a country. Proof of yellow fever vaccination might be required for entry into certain countries for travelers whose itineraries included travel though a yellow fever risk area. For Muslims going on the Haj to Mecca, meningococcal and influenza vaccinations are required.

Each person has a unique profile as to what vaccinations are needed, depending on a variety of variables:

- The age, health, and medical conditions of the traveler and specific allergies
- The travel itinerary, including the countries to be visited, specific regions, and city versus rural
- The purpose and duration of travel
- The anticipated activities (trekking, swimming, animal contact, sexual contact)
- The type of accommodation
- The length of time prior to departure
- Immunizations received previously

For long-term travelers, a TB skin test should be performed prior to departure, and a cholera exemption certificate might be in order depending on location. It is best to visit a travel medicine clinic at least 6 weeks prior to departure to receive all needed vaccinations, as some immunizations come in a series separated by intervals of weeks.

MALARIA PREVENTION

Mosquitoes can be found almost everywhere in the world, and many different species exist. With respect to malaria, only the female anopheles mosquito infects humans with this debilitating and sometimes fatal illness. Both male and female mosquitoes usually feed on fruit and nectar, but the female requires a blood meal every 3 to 4 days to have enough protein to produce eggs.

The anopheles species are dawn and dusk feeders, as opposed to other species that are day feeders. This has significance for protection measures. The low-lying rural and humid areas of the world have the most malaria. Pools of fresh water are where they breed and lay their eggs. Though very humid parts of the world have year-round prevalence, other regions of the world with rainy and dry seasons have a significant increase in disease transmission during and just after the rainy season. The disease can also spread beyond its normal boundaries if a region gets higher than usual rainfall. Migration of peoples with a high infectivity rate can also influence the incidence of the disease. One rarely finds malaria above 6,000–8,000 feet. The global distribution of malarial disease is constantly changing. That is why you need to visit a travel medicine clinic.

Four species of malaria affect humans: *P. falciparum, P. vivax, P. ovale,* and *P. malararie.* The P. falciparum species is the only life-threatening form. However, the P. vivax and P. ovale species can develop up to 3 years after the patient stopped taking chemoprophylaxis. This means that a fever in a returned traveler should always be suspect for malaria. It is crucial to tell your doctor that you have been in a malarial zone within the last 3 years.

Antimalarial medication is prescribed for you at your travel medicine clinic visit if you are going to an area where malaria is present. Your doctor can go over which medication is right for you. Drug resistance exists the world over, and certain malarial prophylaxis medications work better than others in certain parts of the world. Your past medical history and other medications are taken into account, especially seizures and psychiatric illness. The doctor can also go over self-treatment options if you develop a fever and are a distance from definitive medical care. Personal protective measures are crucial because chemoprophylaxis is not always 100% protective. We offer advice on precautions for insect bites in Chapter 8.

MEDICAL KITS FOR GLOBAL HEALTH MISSIONS

Organizing your medical kit prior to your mission requires a little time and effort. You cannot provide for every conceivable accident or illness that might occur. You will always face a struggle between taking the right supplies in the right amounts versus the expense involved and the weight incurred. Excessive supplies and medications make for complex logistics and difficulty in finding particular items when needed quickly.

Serious injuries are thankfully rare. The most common medical problems are blisters, cuts and abrasions, musculoskeletal injuries, insect bites, bowel problems, routine colds and flu, and dental and eye issues. You might also face environment-specific medical problems such as altitude illness, hypothermia, falls in remote environments, sunburn and heat-related illnesses in hot climates, and infectious diseases in jungle areas that require additional supplies and medications. You usually need to take almost as many supplies on a smaller, shorter mission as on a larger one, because the same issues are as likely to occur.

Each member of the mission should carry his or her own small personal medical kit that should include the basic essentials to deal with blisters, allergies, sprains, colds, cough, bites, itching, and low-grade pain. Many preassembled commercial kits are readily available online at a reasonable cost. You should then add to that kit prescription medications and personal supplies that you need. Keep medications in waterproof containers, shielded from light, and clearly labeled. Pack items that might be attractive to thieves, such as needles, syringes, and narcotics, carefully. You must ensure that you can travel with these items legally before packing them.

Prior to your mission, contact the embassy of the country or countries to be visited to ascertain whether or not specific restrictions exist on medications and what paperwork needs to be filed in advance. A letter from your doctor using official letterhead, describing the medications and supplies, can be extremely useful at border crossings. Keep medicines in original labeled containers, and bring a copy of your prescriptions along with the generic names.

Often travelers will hear from others that they should purchase their needed medications at their destination, because they will be much cheaper. However, doing so is hazardous because many cheap medications are counterfeit; your prescription will probably not be available at your destination, or if it is, it might have another name or not come in the same dosages. You should have your prescriptions filled at your local pharmacy and carry everything you need, as you can never be certain you will find it at your destination.

You can find many examples on the Internet or in travel medicine books that describe the contents of what a medical kit should include. Some examples are spartan, while others are probably too extensive. A sample basic kit is as follows:

- **ALLERGIES, BITES, and STINGS:** Antihistamine tablets, epinephrine injection, after-bite gel

- **BLISTERS and SPRAINS:** molefoam, band-aids, splints, and elastic bandages

- **COLD and COUGH SUPPLIES:** Antihistamine caplets, cough suppressant tablets, sore throat relief tablets, decongestant tablets, saline nasal spray

- **CUTS, ABRASIONS, and BURNS:** Adhesive strips, adhesive tape, cotton balls, eye pad and eye drops, hydrocortisone cream, nonadherant pad, antifungal cream, triple antibiotic ointment, tweezers, Xeroform, aloe vera gel

- **DENTAL KIT:** Alcohol preps, acetaminophen tablets, oral antiseptic-anesthetic gel, temporary tooth filling paste such as Tempanol or Cavit, cotton swabs, dental floss, finger cots, salt, oil of cloves

- **FEVER and PAIN SUPPLIES:** Ibuprofen tablets, acetaminophen tablets, thermometer

- **GASTROINTESTINAL TREATMENTS:**
  Antidiarrheal tablets, oral rehydration salts,
  antiemetic/nausea pills, and antacid tablets

- **INFECTION CONTROL:** Sterile gloves, condoms,
  CPR microshield

- **TRAVEL ACCESSORIES:** Insect repellent,
  mosquito net, sunblock, sunglasses, iodine tablets,
  hypothermia blanket, sewing kit with scissors, and
  disinfectant towelettes

- Women of childbearing age must consider supplies
  for menstruation. In most urban settings, tampons
  are available but in rural areas of poorer countries,
  thin pads and tampons may not be available. Female
  travelers might also consider adding medications
  for yeast infections to their medical kit. Menstrual
  hygiene is a concern for women worldwide. For
  more information you may wish to read *Menstrual
  Hygiene* (available at www.eepa.be/wcm/
  dmdocuments/BGpaper_Menstrual-Hygiene.pdf).

EVACUATION INSURANCE

Evacuation insurance is of particular importance to global
health mission members. Most U.S. health insurance plans do
not cover costly repatriation in the event of a serious illness
or injury. Foreign hospitals and doctors expect cash or credit
card payment up front, and you must then submit your bills in
English to your insurance company for reimbursement. Travel
medical insurance that guarantees payment to foreign doctors
and hospitals, as well as air evacuation in case of extreme
emergency, is essential.

One of the most useful aspects of evacuation insurance is that the insurance company can direct you to the nearest English-speaking doctor and begin the process of helping you find the most appropriate place to receive care. Sometimes evacuation is not the answer if you can be treated locally. For example, cases of malaria have been missed in U.S. hospitals, especially if the doctor hasn't asked about foreign travel and you haven't volunteered the information. Doctors at your local destination are accustomed to seeing and treating the local diseases. Most air evacuation is because of trauma and the need for surgery.

Should air evacuation be necessary, it's much easier to have an insurance company work with the air ambulance company to make the arrangements. If the medical condition is serious enough to warrant an air ambulance, the cost is enormous. The insurance company can help with the communication, which includes

- The administrative medical director at the insurance company
- The physician who is caring for the patient overseas
- The logistics support staff
- The repatriation flight team
- The physician at the accepting hospital
- Ambulance companies on both ends
- Translators if necessary
- Airport administration on both ends
- Immediate family members
- Family physician if possible

Make sure the plan you select does not have exemptions for age or preexisting conditions. Some plans cover your evacuation from a major city in the country back to the United States, but do not cover your evacuation from a remote area to the major city, such as from Everest base camp to Kathmandu, or the Serengeti Plain to Nairobi or Dar es Salaam. These helicopter rides can be costly and often require cash up front. Our co-author, Rhonda, spent much time on the satellite phone when she was a medical volunteer in the Himalayas calling parents or friends of injured trekkers to put $5,000 on their credit card so that their loved one could just be flown out to Kathmandu.

Most people believe that infectious diseases are the most common health hazard for those traveling to the developing world when, in fact, it is trauma that is responsible for almost all morbidity and mortality abroad. About one-third of all insurance claims from foreign travelers are medical expenses related to trauma, and more than half of all repatriations are trauma patients. Many travelers fail to use common sense and often take more risks when away from home—participating in dangerous road travel, not using seat belts and helmets, swimming in dangerous areas, and engaging in high-risk sports—often exacerbated by alcohol.

The statistics on road accidents in developing countries are grim. Drivers in all sorts of vehicles from buses to trucks to private cars are often intoxicated and not well-trained, vehicles are poorly maintained, safety regulations are lacking, the roads are often not policed, and many roads have no lighting, guard rails, or other safety features. Therefore, it is no surprise that road accidents account for most traumas abroad.

While traveling abroad, Rhonda encountered marijuana-smoke-infested taxi cabs, buses that ran out of gas in the middle of major roads, impossible-to-cross streets because of cars traveling in all directions with no regard to lanes or traffic lights, sidewalks where she had to compete with cows and rickshaws and that had huge potholes where ankles could easily be twisted or broken, and helmetless motorcycle drivers carrying several passengers on one bike flying by. A distracted traveler can be a dead traveler. We recommend judicious use of local vehicles, particularly small motorcycles, in the poorer countries where their use is not regulated.

SAFETY AND LEGAL ISSUES

As a traveler and global health mission member, you always feel more vulnerable to a host of problems when far from home and family. In many instances, you really are more vulnerable to such problems as crime, exposure to illicit drugs and sexual assault, and certain legal and cultural issues unique to the country where you are traveling or working.

Unless you educate yourself ahead of time about the people, values, religion, and traditions of the region where the mission is going to take place, you run the risk of making mistakes in a variety of areas. Assuming that others share your values, culture, and legal traditions can lead to much unnecessary anguish.

Higher levels of crime often exist in many countries because of significant disparities of income and different value systems. Foreigners are often perceived by locals to be rich as well as vulnerable because they are guests in the country.

Many countries are not as tolerant of those arrested for crimes as you might find in your home country. A lot of countries take a harsh stand on buying and selling drugs. If arrested, you might find yourself living in the grossly substandard conditions of their jails and lacking adequate representation for your rights. Staying away from drugs, alcohol, shady bars, and dubious sex partners is more than prudent.

You need to learn and respect local customs and the local dress code. Recently, a British couple was jailed in the United Arab Emirates for hugging and kissing in public. Public displays of affection are illegal in the Emirates and frowned upon in many other cultures. Women should be especially cautious and respectful about how they dress.

However, even when you are being cautious, problems can occur. Prior to leaving, American citizens should review the travel warnings on the Department of State website and register for their planned travel. It is best to register your presence and purpose at your country's embassy upon arrival. It pays to keep in contact with those at home when possible, giving information as to your whereabouts and activities. Other simple suggestions include

- Dress conservatively; flashy clothes and jewelry put a mark on you as affluent.

- Keep valuables in a safe place and have backup copies of important documents.

- When carrying valuable or important documents on your person, use a pouch or money belt tucked inside your clothes, and try to conceal them in several places instead of a single place. Hidden belts are very helpful.

- Don't go out on beaches at night.

- Don't hitchhike or pick up hitchhikers.

- Book hotel rooms above the second floor to lessen risk of break-ins.

- Avoid politically unstable regions where you might encounter civil unrest.

- Avoid using handbags or loose fitting backpacks.

- Don't use short cuts, alleys, or poorly lit streets.

- Keep a low profile and avoid loud conversations.

- Never discuss travel plans or identify where you are staying to a stranger.

- Beware that pickpockets often have accomplices.

The living quarters where you are assigned might be very crowded, and many times you have no safe place to leave valuables, money, or a computer. These are considerations that you need to work through with the organizations that you have chosen to work with. If you cannot guarantee the safety of your personal belongings, it might be best to leave them at home.

Safety on the street requires the same common sense that you would exercise at home. If at all possible, get good directions from a reliable source before you start out. Try to avoid very crowded, unfamiliar places, such as buses, shared taxis, marketplaces, and marginal areas of a community. Be wary of scams. If you look purposeful as you travel about, you're less likely to be a target of scam artists. If you are offered items for sale that seem just too good to be true, they probably are! This might be a come-on for you to "see" other items located elsewhere. If you become lost, ask directions from people in authority, like policemen or guards at banks. If you have a cell phone that works at your assignment site, have important numbers on speed dial for emergencies.

PLANNING TO COMMUNICATE WITH OTHERS

Many volunteers bring their own laptop computers, but a computer is just one more thing that you would need to protect while on assignment. So, before you travel you can determine if computers are available on-site to which volunteers have access. In addition, you might locate a convenient, inexpensive Internet café where you are assigned. Your parent organization should be able to answer these questions.

You might have international service on your personal mobile or cell phone. You need to investigate the service plan to see what the costs are. In some settings, you can get international service, but the cost is prohibitive. It is often more economical to get a phone in the country where you are assigned. In many countries, cell phones can be purchased for about US $20 and minute cards added as needed. The US $24 that Jeanne spent on her Ugandan phone was well worth it, both as a way to connect with nurses and other colleagues in Uganda and as a way to be reached from home. Though this phone does not work outside of Uganda, Jeanne can use it on each return trip, and it cost her about US $3 per week.

Another option for communication with family and friends back home is to open a Skype account. This works on your personal computer with Internet service. Visit http://www.skype.com/intl/en-us/home to learn about the Internet-based options for telephone calls with web camera options. Both Jeanne and Julie have used this to communicate with others globally. It is helpful to set this up from home.

Additionally, the ability to use Internet services for professional reasons is essential for those volunteers involved in educational service. Many organizations include education of local staff or other professionals such as nurses as part of volunteer service. While some materials can be transported easily on a flash drive, shared with host partners, and printed at the location abroad, circumstances arise where professional colleagues from home can send materials electronically to the volunteer. Increasingly, volunteer organizations seek to provide Internet service to the local staff in the host setting to improve health services even in more remote settings. While Jeanne served with HVO in Uganda, she worked with nursing faculty at Makerere University. During her extended stay, she identified other topics beyond what she had brought along that might be of use to the faculty there. Faculty colleagues at her home university willingly shared their teaching materials, sending them as attached files, and Jeanne was able to share these with the nursing faculty at Makerere.

DECISIONS ABOUT TRAVELING WITH OTHER FAMILY MEMBERS

You might desire to have a family member travel with you. This is sometimes possible if your family member has a particular skill such as fluency in the host country language, other medical training, or other skills deemed useful by the volunteer setting. If a suitable assignment is available at the same site, this situation can be a rewarding experience for you and your family member. However, it can become stressful for the accompanying family members if not enough meaningful work exists for them to do while you are at work. Unless they are going to be involved in a useful project, it is best that they do not come along with you for your volunteer effort.

PACKING FOR THE TRIP

Before you begin packing your suitcases for an assignment, do research on appropriate dress in your assigned country. In Uganda, women wear dresses or skirts for work or in public. Jeanne and Julia bring skirts and tops to wear during their stay, along with a lab coat and identification name tag. For travel and any sightseeing that involves hiking, it would be acceptable to wear some mid-weight nylon convertible pants and shirts that protect against sun and insects as well. Clothing can be washed on location. In some settings, local women earn money by doing laundry for volunteers. Though we encourage you to pack lightly, you might have to bring a number of items along from home that you cannot find in your assignment location. The following packing list is a guide. We suggest that you consult with the organization you plan to travel with to determine what items will be essential and what can be left behind.

PACKING LIST
CLOTHING:

- Skirts
- Pants/shorts for travel
- Sweater or lightweight fleece
- Blouses
- Tee shirts
- Shoes
- Socks
- Bathing suit
- Sun hat
- Bandana

- Scrubs (if required for work)
- Sturdy shoes (work)
- Sandals/flip-flops or shower shoes
- Waterproof shoes
- Underwear
- Pajamas or nightgowns
- Jacket (waterproof, breathable fabric)
- Robe
- Messenger bag
- Umbrella
- Poncho
- Sunglasses
- Bras

PERSONAL:

- Soap, wash cloth, towels
- Toothpaste, toothbrush
- Medical kit
- Sunscreen
- Water purification tablets
- Sun/shower bag
- Book(s) or reading material
- Candle/matches
- Earplugs
- Personal toiletries
- Nail brush/nail file
- Small mirror
- Mosquito net
- Book light
- Duct tape
- Toilet paper roll
- Backpack and reusable tote bags
- Water bottle (non-BPA refillable bottle)
- Insect repellant (with DEET)
- Medications (see suggestions for personal medical kits in text; should be kept in original containers)
- Hair dryer and curling iron may not work where you are traveling, so be sure to check on this before taking them along
- Extra pair of glasses or contact lenses
- Flashlight, reading lamp, or head lamp as electricity might not be reliable
- Small games such as UNO, Canasta, Yahtzee, and cards for other games with volunteers
- MP3 player and charger, camera and battery, memory cards, extra batteries for all items

DOCUMENTATION:

- Passport
- Copy of travel insurance
- 2–6 photocopies of your passport
- Contact information for all travel contacts
- Visa if needed
- Airline tickets

OFFICE SUPPLIES:

- Small pad of paper
- Small pocket calendar
- Permanent marking pens
- Language dictionary
- Markers and pens, scissors, stapler, and a few office-type supplies
- Flash drive
- Handouts
- Textbooks

PROFESSIONAL SUPPLIES:

- Nametag
- Stethoscope
- Otoscope
- 2 lab coats, so you can have one clean at all times
- Medical/nursing/pharmacy references
- Hand sanitizer
- Bandage scissors

POSSIBLE GIFTS FOR NURSE COLLEAGUES:

- Pens (we all enjoy pens)
- Small calendars
- Small hand lotions/creams, soaps
- Any item with your college/university logo
- Simple art supplies for children, stickers for children
- Small hand sanitizers with straps to attach to belts and pockets
- Nice notepads
- Calculators
- Stethoscopes

If you are staying for a long period of time and have to do your own shopping, food preparation, and housecleaning, then you might need the following:

KITCHEN/HOUSEHOLD:

- Hand towels, washcloths, nylon scrubbies for the shower, microfiber towels of several sizes (a must), your own sheets and pillowcases
- Small container of laundry detergent/clothesline
- Set of silverware, paring knife, and a small plastic cereal bowl (I used them for yogurt and with bananas and apples for snacks and lunches.)
- Cloth or canvas shopping bag, in addition to a backpack to carry items on shopping trips
- Kleenex and cloth handkerchiefs
- Hot pads, kitchen towels, and scrubber for dishes
- Powdered drink mixes
- Protein bars or snacks
- Tea bags

ITINERARY AND TRAVEL

Travel can be both exciting and exhausting for the volunteer. For many volunteers who travel abroad, travel involves several flight transfers and land transportation. For those who bring the maximum weight allowed for donations, this can involve logistical issues of how to get heavy luggage from home to the volunteer site. Beyond the details of travel, we also discuss health risks and how to minimize adverse health effects of long trips.

FLIGHT AND TRANSFERS

When you are planning your trip overseas, shop around when buying your airline ticket. Many organizations assist with this or recommend a travel agent that they have used for other volunteers. Your own local travel agent might have access to information and deals to remote areas. If you buy your ticket from your own travel agent or online, getting assistance for an emergency, like a missed flight or cancellation, might be difficult. Some organizations require the assignee to obtain travel insurance. Whether it is required or not, you will find it's a good idea to purchase this type of insurance. If you should become ill while in a foreign country, it is very expensive to be evacuated. Even though it is seldom used, the insurance provides peace of mind for you and your family while you are away. It is a good idea to avoid arriving late at night for security reasons. If this is unavoidable, plan to stay near the airport and travel to your volunteer site the following day.

JET LAG

The effects of jet lag occur because your body's biological clock becomes out of sync with your new time zone at your destination. Symptoms include fatigue, insomnia, and alterations in appetite. Whenever possible, include a layover day of rest for every six time zones crossed. It takes about 24 hours to adjust to each time zone crossed. Do not plan any important meetings in your first 24 hours post-arrival. Melatonin, a hormone supplement found in natural food stores that is derived from the amino acid tryptophan, is sometimes used to help with jet lag, but its efficacy has not been established.

HAZARDS OF AIR TRAVEL

Seasoned travelers recognize that traveling by air creates some risks to health. Some of these occur as a result of exposure to airborne infectious agents inhaled through the recirculated air on aircraft. Recently, airlines have started warning travelers about the risks of deep vein thrombosis (DVT) for those who travel on extended flights of many hours and offer suggestions to reduce the risk of DVT. Here we offer a more extensive discussion to help you reduce your risks during air travel.

Respiratory Infections—Precautions to prevent respiratory infections in other settings apply to air travel. Though infectious agents such as viruses and bacteria can be inhaled, risks from hand contact can be reduced. Use of antibacterial hand sanitizer and good hand-washing techniques are important as preventive strategies to reduce infections acquired during travel to and from the volunteer site. Though the evidence is equivocal, many travelers take Vitamin C or herbal supplements prior to travel in hopes of boosting their immunity to infection.

Blood Clots—The prospect of air travel can provoke fear or frustration with lost luggage, delayed flights, and missed connections. Yet these inconveniences conceal a greater danger shared by all passengers—a deep vein thrombosis (DVT). Though all immobility (4 hours or more) contributes to clot formation, air travel in particular increases the risk. Cabin air pressure is calibrated to 6,000–8,000 feet. At this pressure altitude, the body starts to increase clotting factors in response. Recirculated air on planes is very dry, and lack of humidity and hydration contribute to blood thickening. Alcohol and coffee both accelerate dehydration. Most passengers sit with legs in the dependent position, allowing blood to pool in the lower extremities.

These conditions are often called "coach class syndrome," but this is a misnomer. Clots can occur just as often in first class, and in cars, buses, trains, and even in army tanks, as evidenced by the death of NBC reporter David Bloom in Iraq (Kleber, 2011). Clots can break loose days, or even weeks, after a long flight. If symptoms that are described below occur, you should inform your doctor that you have been on a long air flight. Data varies, but statistics indicate that one air passenger a month dies within minutes to hours after landing at Heathrow airport, London, and that perhaps as many as 400 passengers per year arriving in Sydney, Australia, have a DVT. The number of air passengers is going up yearly, and now more than 2 billion air passengers are flying. With that perspective, the risk is small but the consequences to the individual are serious (Ball, 2003).

Anecdotal evidence suggests that the number of these events occurring might be more than are documented. Stories persist of passengers dying shortly after a flight arrival, with family and friends assuming it was a heart attack or some other unlikely diagnosis. In reality, it was probably a pulmonary embolus. Rhonda witnessed two deaths in the emergency room where she works in Boston. Both passengers had taken nonstop flights from the West Coast.

Risk factors and prevention strategies are now well-known. Risk factors include

- Prolonged immobility, especially with legs dependent
- History of recent fracture, surgery, or serious illness
- Birth control pills or hormone replacement therapy

- Pregnancy
- Obesity
- Advanced age
- History of cancer, stroke, heart failure, diabetes, peripheral vascular disease, or family/genetic history of a clotting disorder

Early symptoms of a DVT are:

- Muscle pain, swelling, or tenderness in the legs
- Discoloration in a painful area

Serious symptoms of a PE are:

- Shortness of breath and worsening chest pain with breathing
- Coughing up blood
- Feeling faint, sweaty, dizzy, or turning blue
- Racing heartbeat

If these symptoms occur, seek immediate medical attention.

The best advice is to prevent DVT. The following are simple but effective preventive measures for deep vein thrombosis:

- Avoid dehydration by drinking water liberally and avoiding alcohol and caffeine
- Get up hourly and walk around
- Do leg exercises at your seat
- Wear compression stockings
- Avoid wearing tight-fitting clothes
- Discuss with your doctor about taking aspirin

Finally, we remind you that preparation for your volunteer assignment involves dealing with logistical, social, cultural, and health promotion issues. To adequately prepare for your assignment, you must learn about the location and the people who live there. In particular you need to study the history, politics, and culture to better understand the relationship between their everyday lives and their health and illness. Hopefully, this includes reading at least one book about the people you are going to work with. You should learn about 50–100 useful words in the language most commonly spoken where you are going to volunteer. You must prepare for your professional role and be sure to learn about conditions endemic in the area where you plan to serve. If you are traveling abroad, begin your preparations early and start the packing process early enough to have all essential items in advance of your departure. You should have all documents prepared, and ensure that your passport is current for at least 6 months past your return home date and that you have other documentation such as your visa, nursing license, travel insurance, flight information, and important travel contact information. This information should be duplicated, so that you have copies of each document. You should have your health and safety plans completed, including immunizations, prophylactic medications, and your emergency medical kit and protective equipment. Pack your medications in resealable plastic bags to avoid leakage, and be sure to keep them in original packages. Most important is that you feel ready for your assignment. After all your preparations are made, you can enjoy the anticipation of the new experience that awaits you.

BECOMING AN EFFECTIVE VOLUNTEER

- Plan early to make application for your assignment.

- Consider the expenses incurred by the volunteer.

- Identify ways to reduce your personal expenses through scholarships or donations.

- If appropriate to your assignment, find ways to solicit monetary and nonmonetary donations.

- Attend to professional licensure and certification issues for professional practice.

- Learn about assessment and management of the common health problems encountered in the host location.

- Learn about the history, politics, and culture of your host location.

- Learn 50 common words used in the host location.

- Prepare for your health needs: Visit a travel clinic and prepare your personal medical kit.

- Obtain travel insurance.

- Consider safety and legal issues unique to the volunteer setting.

- Make arrangements to communicate with colleagues and loved ones at home.

- Pack wisely.

- Consider your travel needs and plan wisely.

CHAPTER 8

ON ASSIGNMENT

–with Rhonda Martin

Finally the time has come, and you arrive at your volunteer destination. For some of you, it might be the end of a trip across your own country to a disaster or other location. For many of you reading this book, you arrive in an airport in a distant country, where you immediately become aware that you have left home. Beginning with your departure from the airplane, you are likely to see vast differences in the airport routine. Passing through immigration, locating your baggage, and proceeding through customs can be tedious and stressful. Behaviors that you observe at the airport might cause you to be fearful (Heuer & Bengiamin, 2001). After you arrive outside the customs hall, the chaos and confusion are often overwhelming, as you must fend off people trying to take your bags, hoping that they will be paid to help you carry your luggage. It is always helpful to have a firm plan about where to meet your hosts or where to find the local transportation, so you can depart the airport efficiently.

ARRIVAL

In many locations you have to spend your first night somewhere in the arrival city, because the time to travel to your volunteer site is too long and travel in the dark of night is too unsafe. As you travel to your housing for the first night, you will experience many new sights, sounds, and smells that totally immerse you into the experience. This sudden immersion can cause feelings of excitement, fear, curiosity, anxiety, anticipation, and discomfort all at the same time. In addition you are likely to be tired, depending upon the length of time you have traveled from your home to the host country.

No matter how much you prepare before your immersion into the new setting, the differences in location, culture, language, and setting will have a profound effect upon you when you finally arrive at your destination. In this chapter we offer suggestions from our own experiences and those of other nurse colleagues to help you make adjustments to your living and work settings. We discuss factors involved in settling into the new location, making accommodations to your housing, respecting the local culture, working with others, and dealing with the unexpected. Our best advice is to be open to the new experience without allowing the fears or anxieties to overwhelm your emotions. Recognize that the new surroundings, people, language, customs, and experience will become familiar within a few days. It is best to accept these feelings as normal and use whatever strategies help you make adjustments to any significant changes.

The experience for each volunteer, and for each assignment, whether it is your first time or a subsequent visit, differs for a variety of reasons. Personnel and leadership might change at the volunteer site, living conditions might change, and the focus of the assignment can vary. So, whether you are a new or experienced volunteer, this chapter can offer you information to help you during your volunteer experience. In the sidebar below, Pamela Llewellyn of the United Kingdom shares some wisdom from her experiences volunteering abroad.

CHANGING LIVES

During the early days of my placement as a VSO volunteer, I encountered a few difficulties. I thought that I had prepared myself as much as possible, but not everything went according to plan. There were unforeseen challenges and frustrations, and as a result, I felt lonely and isolated. Through determination and encouragement from others, I stayed and enjoyed 2 very happy and fulfilling years.

- *The job you go out to do may only exist on paper and is not actually achievable by anybody. Some volunteers throw in the towel early while others, determined to remain, stand back and ask what job can be done that is achievable. The ability to think sideways is a great asset.*

- *Take care of your health. During the first 6 months of my placement, I lost a lot of weight. My diet had changed drastically, and I felt quite stressed. Some volunteers neglect their malaria prophylaxis, whilst others find comfort in cheap alcohol. It's a vulnerable time. Eventually I became creative with cooking root vegetables and began to grow more familiar salad vegetables in my own garden patch. Cooking for others made it a bigger challenge and more fun. My homemade bread was probably pretty awful, but everyone loved it.*

- *Whilst VSO's training programme in the UK is excellent, the in-country language-training programme is minimal. Be prepared to do some serious local language training. A little goes a long way. Not only does it enable you to communicate better, it also demonstrates a willingness to be part of a new community, and my efforts were much appreciated by local people.*

- *Volunteering overseas, on a new continent and in a new culture, especially in rural areas, can be a very lonely experience. No electricity, no television, etc., can make for lots of lonely nights and weekends. I had to find strategies for entertaining and looking after myself. Above all I had to find a circle of friends that I could socialise with and turn to in "emergencies" or on low days.*

- *Any visitor to any foreign country in the world is vulnerable. I felt safe most of the time but soon came to realise that the very poor society that I was living and working in saw me as "a rich muzungu." Every day I was approached for money, small sums and big, and it takes awhile to decide how, if at all, I was going to handle this. No doubt some of the stories were true and others less so. Sometimes there was obvious need, but I couldn't give to everybody.*

- *Try to enjoy this unique opportunity to be immersed into a new culture. This became the thing that I valued most about my volunteering experience. By accepting invitations to weddings, burials, and into peoples' homes and churches, I made some very wonderful friends and felt privileged to be there.*

(Pamela Llewellyn, personal communication, 2010)

SETTLING INTO THE NEW ENVIRONMENT

If it is your first visit to a foreign country, you will face some degree of culture shock, which can be a challenging experience. Culture shock is often defined as conflict that you feel or the emotions you experience when traveling or living in a culture different from your own (Collins, DeZerega, & Heckscher, 2002; Heuer & Bengiamin, 2001). While we may not always be aware of our own culture and the cultural expectations incorporated into our beings and daily lives, we all are shaped by expectations that we believe are normal or basic to all people. Upon entry and immersion into a new culture (both at home and abroad), we find we are no longer familiar with the daily routine, the expectations, and the way of life of our hosts. Culture shock refers to the impact you might feel when you enter a culture very different from one to which you are accustomed. No matter how well you are prepared, you encounter many things in a culture that you cannot find in books. Differences in nonverbal communication and unwritten rules of behavior are often new and confusing to you. Culture shock can occur on short trips or long trips and to seasoned travelers who are facing a new experience or to first-time travelers. The close and personal experience of poverty, harsh living conditions, unfamiliar food options, lack of simple amenities such as electricity and clean water, and lack of privacy and personal space can be overwhelming for some individuals, especially as the days go on and fatigue sets in. The University of Wisconsin Center for Global Health (2009) describes manifestations of culture shock (see Table 8.1) that may (but not always) include some of the following signs and symptoms.

TABLE 8.1

**SIGNS AND SYMPTOMS OF CULTURE SHOCK
(CENTER FOR GLOBAL HEALTH, 2009)**

Frustration	Irritability
Hypersensitivity	Overreacting
Mental fatigue	Boredom
Lack of motivation	Physical discomfort
Over-concern for cleanliness	Loss of perspective
Disorientation about how to work with/relate to others	
Suspicion (feeling like everyone is trying to take advantage of you)	

Feelings can vary from moments of elation at meeting new people to irritation. The Center for Global Health suggestions for dealing with culture shock describe common reactions. "Typical reactions include assuming the problem lies in everyone else (something is wrong with 'them' not 'us'), over-valuing our own culture, defining our culture in moral terms (natural, rational, civilized, polite), under-valuing the new culture and seeing it as immoral, and stereotyping in an attempt to make the world predictable" (Center for Global Health, 2009). Small annoyances in the beginning can become major aggravations later. Some people experience homesickness, hostility toward the new culture, or even physical symptoms, but for most it is simply moments of confusion, discomfort, and adjustment. While these feelings are common responses to the change in culture, they can sometimes lead to examples where volunteers can exhibit cultural insensitivity and inappropriate behavior.

The experts at the Center for Global Health (2009) also warn that the Internet can serve as an unintended source of public sharing of thoughts that disparage those in other cultures. What may be intended as communication to friends and family is often viewed by others and can cause cultural misunderstandings. Therefore, all volunteers should be cautious in their use of blogs, e-mail, YouTube, social networking sites, and print materials that may not reflect positively upon the hosts where we volunteer.

Being aware of the reality of culture shock helps you prepare to learn more about the culture of the place where you will volunteer and effective ways to deal with it when it occurs. Even veteran volunteers can experience culture shock in a new setting. Awareness of the phenomenon can also lead to better adjustment, the patience to allow time to learn and adjust, and the ability to become an effective volunteer and partner to your hosts.

DEALING WITH CULTURE SHOCK

Generally, people adapt to culture shock gradually. You need to avoid making judgments of the experience too quickly as this initial discomfort, in whatever way you experience it, is likely to improve within a few days. As you become more comfortable in the new setting, you will see more of the positive and joyful aspects of living and working in a new cultural environment. Many of the smaller problems can be prevented from becoming larger problems by self-awareness, enthusiasm, and cooperation. The best way to overcome culture shock is to accept that every culture has its own way of understanding things, and your adjustment comes with time. Here are a few strategies to help with this adjustment:

- Talk with seasoned volunteers traveling with you.
- Attend a local church or other public event, such as market day.
- Try to learn more about the daily lives of your host partners.

- Enjoy a meal in a local restaurant.

- Enjoy the local music.

- Spend time with the local children. They can bring joy.

- Keep a private journal of your thoughts for reflection.

- Get adequate rest to help you feel your best physically.

- Focus upon why you chose to volunteer to bring back positive energy.

- Try to live in the moment and realize that time helps you adjust.

Some organizations have an in-country coordinator who can be very helpful to you as you settle into your housing accommodation. As mentioned in Chapter 2, this situation can be vastly different from what you are accustomed to at home. In most instances the sponsoring organization arranges the living accommodations, which can be on-site or at a nearby location. These are as varied as one can imagine: tents, tukuls, dormitory-style rooms, hostels, shared apartments, nurses' residences attached to hospitals, and even local hotels. By talking with the sponsoring organization, you can probably be made more aware in a general way what to expect before you arrive, or you can even view photos posted on a website or through personal communication with previous volunteers. Still, it is common for new volunteers to be surprised by the simple housing available, despite seeing photos or reading about it. Bunkhouses and dormitories can often appear brighter, cleaner, and more inviting in the photos you see prior to your arrival. Again, being open to the experience is our best advice, and generally within a night or two the bunk, dormitory, or tent becomes your home.

RESPECTING LOCAL CULTURE

During this transition from your own home culture into the host country setting, you need to be mindful of the host patterns and country etiquette. Respect the culture of the individuals with whom you are working as you carry out your assignment. They might have preconceived ideas about foreigners from past experiences, ideas that are not flattering. They might consider visitors as arrogant or unfriendly, bringing attitudes of "my way is the best way" or "my way is the only way." Give your new colleagues some time to get to know you. Trust must be established and not presumed. This involves ensuring that your dress, conversation, and behavior make impressions upon those you work with that will be positive, not negative. Be aware of the importance of your nonverbal communication, your manner of dress, your silent reactions in new situations, and your body language, which might not be interpreted in the new situation the same way it is at home. You do not want to insult the host partner's religion or culture by your dress or behavior. You must recognize that your ability to volunteer is a privilege and that to your host partners you appear privileged, despite the fact that you might not be wealthy by your home country standards (Collins, DeZerega, & Heckscher, 2002). In many countries women must wear skirts or dresses and cannot wear pants; men must bring long pants.

Though you might find the dormitory lacking in what you consider comforts of home, the accommodations are generally better than those of most of the population where you volunteer. Having a bathroom in your bunkhouse or dormitory is a luxury, despite the fact that the toilets must be flushed with buckets of water or the showers offer only cold water. Complaining about the accommodations is not respectful to the host partners (Myriam Jeannis, personal communication, January 2011). Most nurse volunteers we speak with are happy to live in simpler housing while on a volunteer assignment, because the enormous disparity between a modern hotel and the homes of those served causes too much psychological confusion for the volunteer.

In addition, how we communicate with others can show disrespect to our hosts. We are guests, and we must afford our hosts respect by acting as the professionals that we are as nurses. We represent not only ourselves but the organization with which we volunteer, our own nursing profession, those institutions we work for at home, and our home country as well. As with all professional communication, we should respect that our hosts deserve the same right to privacy as do patients and clients in our home settings. This right to privacy includes confidential experiences, taking photographs without permission and clear explanation of how those photos will be used, and communicating personal information in public venues (Center for Global Health, 2009).

WORKING WITH OTHERS

You learn to work collaboratively with your nursing colleagues, with other health professionals, and with all of your coworkers early in your nursing education program. This background holds you in good stead when you accept a volunteer assignment and becomes even more significant when away from your home situation. It's usually a good idea to spend the first bit of time observing how things are done in the new environment. The culture of the population affects the way procedures are accomplished. Even though you might think your way is better or more current, learn their way first before making any suggestions. They might have valid reasons for their actions. More likely than not, the lack of available resources dictates many situations. For example, teaching advanced life support using a defibrillator that you have brought with you is a waste of time if the location has no reliable source of electricity and batteries are not readily available. Your time might be better spent reviewing basic life support if this has not been taught recently, rather than in instructing a few nurses or students in the use of equipment that cannot be maintained.

In the sidebar below, Petra Frankhuizen explains that her lack of knowledge of the caste system in Nepal led to confusion and frustration in her assignment.

CHANGING LIVES

Working in an outreach program in Nepal, I had to deal with the caste system. I thought that surely the NGO I worked for had the policy that everybody was treated the same. Therefore, our patients were triaged according to the severity of their illness, and the members of our national staff had to help out if someone else was very busy. I was the outreach supervisor and had various responsibilities. One of them was the transfer of seriously ill patients to the hospital. When I went for holiday, I asked the health advisor (not a medical doctor, but able to do consultations) to cover this job. We had a national staff female doctor, but she had to take care of the female consultations. The man I asked was very capable and had shown interest and knowledge. I had explained who was taking over the responsibility to all the team before I left. Everybody agreed, or so it seemed. But when I returned, I found the team in disagreement; in my absence, they fought, and the whole cooperative team spirit disappeared. I did not understand at all. As it turned out, I had asked a lower caste and not the doctor to do a job they thought the doctor had to fulfill, but nobody dared to tell me so (Petra Frankhuizen, personal communication, 2011).

Despite the extensive preparations you might make to become an effective volunteer, unforeseen situations always occur. We find that following the principles of listening to your host partners, showing respect, and being truly open to learning from your hosts is the most effective path to success. As Greg Mortenson notes in *Three Cups of Tea* (Mortenson & Relin, 2006), you first move from being strangers, to friendship, and finally to family with each successive cup of tea. This refers to the fact that the helper cannot presume to know what is best for those being helped without spending sufficient time getting to know them by first listening to them. Mortenson also states, "The best decisions I make are not about me but about others. My father always told me that your faith is about actions and not about words. It's about listening to people and, instead of helping people, empowering people. There's a big difference between helping and empowering people" (Mortenson, 2011). (Editor's Note: As this book was going to press in April 2011, reports surfaced that Greg Mortenson may have misreported events in his books regarding his travels and work in Afghanistan. In absence of definitive answers, readers may note that his work with the Central Asia Institute continues and has been influential in the region.)

YOUR EVERYDAY WORK AND LEISURE

You are likely to become oriented to your everyday work routine after a short time. However, at first you are likely to feel very tired at the end of the day, not only from a day of hard work but in response to all the new things you see and learn. Additionally, using the language of your host partners, if it is not your primary language, can be tiring. We urge you to make sure you allow time to relax and to get adequate rest. Though this rest is sometimes impossible in emergency or disaster settings, you cannot be effective if you do not take care of your physical and emotional needs. In some settings, we have enjoyed visiting the local markets, restaurants, and cultural events on days when we were not at work. In addition, some volunteers have planned to add a few days or more to their stay to tour or vacation in other areas of the host country. Getting to know your host partners in more relaxed settings outside of the volunteer worksite can also be revitalizing, as well as a way to build relationships. In the sidebar below, Clare Lawrence of the United Kingdom offers tips for volunteers from her volunteer experience.

CHANGING LIVES

Clare Lawrence, a nurse volunteer with VSO, offers these tips for nurse volunteers:

- *Bring with you photos of family, friends, and home to show new colleagues. This helps get conversation going, helps allow others to get to know you, and gives everyone a sense of shared information. Laminate them first, to prevent damage.*

- *Always take a book, the newspaper, or magazines for something else to do when attending meetings, as they almost never start on time!*

- *Learn at least a few words of the local language, and make sure you greet people properly when meeting them.*

- *Set your boundaries. Make sure you have personal time for relaxing and reflecting on your experiences. Writing a blog or journal helps to organize your thoughts and will be interesting to reread later when you've forgotten what it was like at the beginning!*

- *Be content with the small changes that happen. You won't change the world yourself; in fact, you might not even see the effect you've had. But just by volunteering you are contributing something, and that is important (Clare Lawrence, personal communication, 2010).*

EXPECTATIONS

Realism might set in soon after you begin your assignment. Nurses and other health professionals sometimes believe that they can "save the world." We are good, but we need to be realistic. As a volunteer you are there to help, sometimes to provide care, to teach, to share some new ideas, and to learn. Even in some long-term assignments, 6 months to a year, you can hope to accomplish only so much.

If you and the organization have developed your assignment carefully with the receiving site, considering your expertise and experience and the needs of the site, you should have a good idea what you will be doing during your time on-site, be it providing direct service in a clinic or hospital; teaching, either formally or informally; mentoring of students or practicing nurses; or offering consultation to nursing or health organizations. As a volunteer in many situations, Julia found it best to spend the first few days observing how things were being done in the host setting. Tasks can be accomplished in so many ways, and the local nurses have been doing these tasks in a certain way for many years. Only after you realize why procedures are carried out in a particular way can you begin to introduce other possibilities or small changes for accomplishing the tasks, perhaps with increased safety and less effort.

In an upcoming sidebar, Pamela Llewellyn, a VSO volunteer in Masindi, Uganda, explains the importance of making assessments before carrying out your own volunteer plans.

CHANGING LIVES

The burden of disease is high, and there's a burial in most villages most weeks. Often it is for a child less than 5 years old. Malaria, diarrhea, and coughs are the main problems. The government has responded by introducing health care units, trying to bring health care closer to the people, especially in rural areas. Each parish in Miirya now has a health centre that holds daily clinics and special sessions for immunisation and antenatal care. They are now an accepted service, although some patients will have walked for more than 2 hours to get there. The very sick, the very old, and the very poor remain in their villages and often resort to traditional medicine or just die.

The Government Health Decentralisation Policy also advocates the use of community health volunteers to promote health and prevent disease in the villages where they live. Miirya Sub County had attempted to set up village health teams in the past but was not successful. Volunteers had become demotivated and the initiative collapsed. This is where it was hoped that I could make a difference as a community nurse.

THE MIIRYA VILLAGE VOLUNTEER PROJECT

The initial challenge was to find out why past volunteers had become demotivated and inactive. Who were these people and how would I find them, hidden away in 42 villages? I need not have worried. Communication in sub-Saharan Africa is easier than you would think. A combination of radio announcements and the Bush Telegraph worked liked magic. Dates and locations were set for three parish meetings, and I didn't really know what to expect. They came in droves, some on foot, others three to a bicycle, one on a motorcycle. Clearly they did not know what to expect either, and I think some were shocked to see this white old woman (WOW) in front of them. I was the first white nurse to go as a volunteer to Miirya.

The start was tentative and nervous on both sides, but soon the volunteers were eager to air their frustrations, disappointments, and hopes for the future as health care workers. Their commitment remained solid, but they clearly needed nurturing. They felt neglected, uncoordinated, and poorly supported in their roles. Most of the volunteers had considerable knowledge despite not having completed secondary education, even primary in some cases. They asked for training, inclusion at meetings, and recognition through a voice and a uniform. The agenda for the next 2 years was being spelled out. All I had to do was to make it happen!

(Pamela Llewellyn, personal communication, 2010)

After volunteering in Turkish villages for several months, Julia and her nurse colleagues were invited to the home of one of the village women. They observed no running water in the home, even for hand washing. From a nearby airbase they collected discarded 5-gallon jerricans, bought small spigots for very little money, and the husband of one of the volunteers soldered the spigots to the bottoms of the cans. This small change gave the opportunity to teach the importance of running water for hand washing, especially when caring for their children or when in contact with someone who was ill. It was a win-win situation and very well accepted by the village women. We use this example to illustrate the importance of taking the time to observe how and why procedures are done in a particular way. It might inspire you to suggest small changes that can ease the burden on the individuals you are working with. These small changes might eventually lead to system changes in the institution.

Always remember that change is incremental and sometimes very slow. Change does not occur in a short period of time. Sometimes it takes several visits over an extended period of time before you see change. In the sidebar below, Linda Bauman, PhD, RN, FAAN, offers advice for working internationally.

CHANGING LIVES

Over the past 20 years, I have been involved in international nursing in developing countries, mainly Uganda and Vietnam. My first significant experience was serving as a consultant to the Democratic Republic of Vietnam to upgrade skills of nurse teachers and administrators in 1989. For many Americans at that time, Vietnam was a war, not a country. I wasn't prepared for the culture shock during my first visit, and I found that disorienting. I got dehydrated and had multiple bouts of a "bad stomach." My mentor on this first visit gave me invaluable pearls of advice about working internationally that I would like to share.

LINDA'S PEARLS

1. **Never Promise What You Cannot Deliver.** *I thought this was a somewhat simple rule that would not be a problem to comply with; however, I found that over the years this has been the greatest challenge. Part of the challenge in making promises is that the needs are so great. When*

we met with local nursing associations or schools to offer assistance, the list was already prepared: a motorbike, a photocopy machine, funds to attend an international meeting. In medical tourism and international nursing, initial enthusiastic delegations visit needy areas to establish a project, usually with bags of donations that are nonspecific and may be totally useless. A Ugandan colleague who helps to arrange interdisciplinary health science student immersion experiences in community health finds that, despite the initial enthusiasm, most international exchanges do not last more than 3 years, and she's arranged hundreds. I've seen many people coming with enthusiasm to plan a project, only to never return for the real thing.

2. **Begin Where They Are At.** *Fit into the needs of the host country, not your own. Sometimes the initial match is not what you are looking for, but with patience and a commitment that you will return, you will have an opportunity to do what fits your interests. I have been a nurse practitioner in primary care and a community health nurse most of my career. Yet in Vietnam in 1989, nurses worked in hospitals, where most health care was delivered, so I began working with hospital nurses. Only 10 years later, as a result of continued communications and contacts with Vietnamese Nurses Association partners, was I invited to teach and do research with nurses in outpatient care and health education, my areas of expertise.*

3. **Aspire to Maintain a Long-Term Partnership.** *A successful partnership requires mutual respect, cultural humility, and fostering personal relationships. In Uganda, I was able to partner with physicians and nurses who were conducting a national training for teams of health care workers to manage diabetes in district hospitals. This partnership met*

my research and teaching interests and helped to enhance the training conducted by the Ugandan team. Conducting research without Ugandans taking a lead role would have been foolish, since negotiating cultural issues is complex in this setting. Take language, for example. The official language of Uganda is English, yet there are more than 40 tribal languages spoken in the country. In the rural setting we worked in, Luganda was the predominant language, but not everyone spoke this. Further, when we used English in the questionnaires, many participants could not read, either because of low literacy or because they had blurred vision and no corrective lenses. We resolved the language issue by presenting in Luganda and completing questionnaires in a group setting, with staff to assist with reading the English questionnaires to participants. Once the study was completed, we translated the training materials into Luganda and English, yet not everyone would be able to read this language.

Nurses who work internationally have much to offer and much to learn. To be successful requires common goals, sensitivity, hardiness, and a sense of awe about the power of global partnerships to improve health (Linda Baumann, personal communication, 2010).

Another example of a sustained volunteer effort is Julia's experience in Romania. Following the fall of communism in 1990, many atrocities of the system, especially as experienced by children in Romania, were revealed. One of these injustices that made world headlines was the orphanage situation involving 125,000 children living in orphanages primarily because their parents, who were encouraged by the government to produce children, could not provide for them. Julia was assigned to Romania in 1990 to work with the Ministry of Health to improve the care that was provided to the orphans. Careful assessment with Ministry of Health personnel indicated that the caregivers in orphanages had no training in the care of children, and that the orphanages did not have adequate staff or resources to care for these children. Early in this assignment, it came to light that nursing as a profession in Romania was discontinued in 1976. The government had decided that a high school education was sufficient, and that young graduates of high school would be assigned to work in hospitals and learn by observing those people working in the hospital. It seemed these two situations were connected. Without educated nurses to train caregivers, the situation in the orphanages would not change.

By locating several nurses who had been educated before 1976, Julia formed a small working group to address both situations. A proposal was written and submitted by the government to the World Bank to establish nursing schools throughout the country. Although a statistically appropriate number of nursing schools in Romania would have been 8, the proposal the Romanian nurses presented asked for 42 nursing schools—one for each district in the country. Money was secured from the World Bank to establish the schools, and consultants were provided by the World Health Organization to work with the Romanian nurses to develop the curriculum. The consultants worked with the Romanian nurses for 18 months and developed a standardized curriculum.

That 4-month assignment in 1990 became a partnership with Julia's Romanian colleagues that lasted for about 16 years. From 1991 to the present day, many nurses have volunteered their time to assist in reestablishing nursing as a profession. Nursing faculty from the United States, United Kingdom, Denmark, and other countries became involved in Romanian nursing faculty development. Early childhood educators from these countries provided training for the orphanage staff, and Peace Corps volunteers were assigned throughout the country to assist in the development of health and sanitation projects.

The nurses who had been educated before 1976 were very interested in forming a professional organization. Before 1976, the Romanian Nurses Association had been a member of the International Council of Nurses, and once again they were qualified to join their nursing colleagues. During the 16 years of her involvement with the Romanian nurses, Julia volunteered 26 times. Often these visits were self-funded; other times funding came from governmental, faculty, and nongovernmental groups eager to participate in Romanian nursing development. The Romanian Nurses Association is again a member of the International Council of Nurses, and Julia continues to provide consultation and friendship to her colleagues, mainly by e-mail and sometimes by telephone. Having this unique opportunity to serve in this sustained way has been a most rewarding experience for her.

DEALING WITH EMERGENCIES

Any traveler must be vigilant about health and safety when in a setting away from home. In this section we discuss safety issues for food and water, precautions to prevent illness, problems related to hazardous bites from insects and animals, prevention and management of traveler's diarrhea, dental emergencies, and safe sex prophylaxis. The information we provide will be helpful for any traveler, whether traveling to volunteer or for pleasure.

FOOD AND WATER SAFETY

Another new cultural experience might occur when mealtime comes. If it is a large established site, meals might be well organized and eaten with other volunteers. If you are on a solo volunteer assignment, meals might be haphazard—whatever is available on that day—a quick sandwich, a piece of fruit, or some cooked dish. At most sites, meals are supplied as part of the program. Generally, this food is prepared by local cooks and is typical of the diet of the culture of the volunteer site. For example, rice and beans are commonly eaten at midday and dinner every day when you volunteer in many Latino cultures, such as the Dominican Republic. But the staple of rice and beans can be as varied and tasty as the range of cooks who prepare it for you! Remember, though, it is your responsibility to protect your personal health when it comes to food and water.

Many of us are privileged to presume that we will have safe food and water. We have regulations and standards for the companies that produce, process, and package our food. We have refrigerators and preservatives. Regulations govern the purification and sanitation of our water supply and how sewerage is handled. But there are few regulations governing the sanitation of food and water in many parts of the world. Toilets might drain into sources of drinking water; farms are contaminated with various bacteria from human and animal feces; regulations about how restaurants prepare and cook food are nonexistent; and sources of contamination are greater. The resulting lack of hygiene leads to illnesses such as diarrhea, hepatitis A, typhoid fever, polio, and other parasites. Cooking food thoroughly and boiling or purifying water can help to eliminate most of these problems. Food contamination can come from the source, from handling food with dirty hands or utensils, from bacterial growth, or from parasitic larvae in or on the food.

Food poisoning most commonly occurs in the adventurous traveler who samples local cuisine at roadside stands and open-air bazaars or who tries to live off the land. Local herb teas, which are popular, might contain anticholinergic compounds and other unknown substances. Try to wash your hands with soap and water before eating or use hand sanitizer liberally. Carrying a bottle of sanitizer or packaged wipes with you at all times is a good idea. The safest drinks to have are bottled carbonated drinks, hot tea or coffee, beer, wine, boiled water, or water that has been treated with iodine or chlorinated tablets. Plan to bring your own drinking water to your work site every day.

It is probably best to eat only cooked foods, including vegetables, meat, or fish. If you are doing your own food preparation, you should shop for locally grown fresh fruits and vegetables to avoid food that might have spoiled in transport. Meat and fish should be thoroughly cooked. Canned and prepared foods tend to be more expensive and not as healthy as fresh food, rice, and locally baked goods. While Jeanne was in Uganda staying at the Health Volunteers Overseas apartment at the Mulago Guest House, she shared shopping and cooking with several other volunteers. This arrangement reduced the time spent on chores and allowed for shared expenses and the enjoyment of group dining.

The most important rule for eating is, "Boil it, cook it, peel it, or forget it!"

Here are some other precautions:

- Avoid cold cuts, salads, and watermelons.

- Avoid raw shellfish and uncooked meat and fish.

- Avoid unpasteurized milk and dairy products, including cheese.

- Avoid sauces and condiments, especially at room temperature.

- Eat food that has been thoroughly cooked and served hot.

- Avoid consuming food purchased from street vendors.

- Avoid eating raw fruits and vegetables unless they can be peeled.

- Do not purchase fruits that have been cut, because a dirty knife can contaminate even peeled fruit or vegetables.

WATER

As with food, water in less developed countries should be considered unsafe. Filtered and chlorinated tap water might be safe in some cities, hotels, and resorts. Mission groups need to review in advance what their water needs will be, where they plan to obtain it, and how they plan to sterilize it. Some settings will provide bottled water and encourage volunteers to keep a 1- to 2-quart refillable water bottle filled at all times. The ideal water container for an individual is a wide mouth Nalgene or stainless steel refillable bottle. In tropical climates, the importance of maintaining hydration cannot be overemphasized. In some settings, if you are responsible for personal cooking and drinking, you need to boil water for at least 1 minute to ensure that all harmful microorganisms are destroyed. In Zaire (now the Democratic Republic of the Congo) after the Rwandan genocide, only large military units had the ability to purify and desalinate water for thousands of refugees and displaced persons. As a volunteer, you should carry water-purifying tablets for personal use, as clean water is a precious commodity in many places.

You need to ask these questions:

- What environment will you be in and for how long?
- Will you be storing drinking water in a vehicle, and how many containers can you carry?
- How many are in your group, and how much water needs to be sterilized at one time?
- How close will you be to sources of water?
- What illnesses are common at your destination?
- What type of sterilization equipment will be taken?

Use these general rules for avoiding unsafe water:

- Avoid tap water, mixed drinks, ice cubes, and local alcohol.
- Avoid locally bottled and uncapped bottled water.
- Sea water is not safe to drink, but can be used for cooking.
- Even pristine-looking water might harbor unsafe organisms.
- Don't brush your teeth with tap water. If you do so accidently, use a new toothbrush (bring extras with you).
- Don't open your mouth in the shower.

INSECT PRECAUTIONS AND HAZARDOUS BITES

The mosquito transmits malaria, yellow fever, Japanese encephalitis, dengue fever, and West Nile virus. Even though vaccines and medications help prevent some of these illnesses, your first line of defense is personal protective measures that prevent bites in the first place. In some cases, such as dengue fever, no vaccine or medication is currently available.

Dengue is the most common arbovirus in man, comprising about 40 million cases worldwide annually. The virus is spread by the day-biting Aedes mosquito, which breeds in clean water. The incubation period is 2 to 7 days. Classical dengue causes fever and muscle aches and has a characteristic measles-like rash. The illness lasts for about a week and is seldom fatal. Illness confers immunity to further attacks of the same serotype, but not to others. The dangerous variant is dengue hemorrhagic fever (DHF). It provokes a breakdown in the blood clotting system, which can result in bleeding and shock. This form is seen in Southeast Asia and the Pacific region. Travelers to countries in the Western Hemisphere are at low risk for DHF. Prevention includes all the usual mosquito bite preventive measures. No vaccine is available at this time.

Swimming in fresh water in many regions of the world can expose you to a blood fluke infection called shistosomiasis. You should avoid swimming and wading in slow-moving freshwater lakes, rivers, and streams. If contact with water is unavoidable, towel rub your skin immediately afterward to remove any possible parasites.

Many species of worms, sand flies, and ticks also pose potential hazards. The best way to avoid these is by wearing closed footwear and protective clothing tucked into footwear and by using insecticides containing DEET.

Snakebites are very rare but can occur in many rural regions of Africa and Asia. The risk increases if you are living and working in these areas and have living conditions similar to the local population. Most snakes hunt at night in grassy areas. Walking at night in high-risk areas should be avoided. Wearing appropriate footwear and making shuffling noises when walking warns the snake of your presence and likely makes it run away. If you, or a colleague, are bitten, follow these steps:

- Avoid panic.
- Try to identify the offending species of snake.
- Immobilize the bitten extremity by splinting.
- Obtain medical assistance and seek antivenom.
- Clean the wound thoroughly, but don't incise or suck the wound.
- Give acetaminophen for pain, but not aspirin.

Use these personal protective measures:

- Wear clothes that are light-colored (white when possible) and shirts and pants that have long sleeves or are adjustable to full-length.
- Stay as covered as possible between dusk and dawn. Trouser bottoms can be tucked into socks or boots, and there should be tight cuffs on shirts/blouses.
- Clothes should be sprayed with an insect repellent containing permethrin. It should be applied before you put on your clothes, and ideally your clothes should be of a tight weave.
- Use an insect repellent containing DEET on exposed skin and reapply every 12 hours, or more often, as needed. Apply sunscreen 30 minutes prior to repellent.

- Sleep in air-conditioned quarters or under a mosquito net impregnated with permethrin (reapply every 6 months) and inspected for holes, and possibly use vaporizing coils, if available, near the bed.

- Wear boots and socks, not sandals.

- Your living quarters should be sprayed well with insecticide to keep out poisonous spiders, which tend to bite at night, as well as a host of other insects.

- Sleeping under a mosquito net is crucial for not only malaria prevention, but also to keep any and all pests away while sleeping.

- Avoid using scented soaps or perfumes.

SUN SAFETY

Unsafe exposure to the sun is a concern not only for nurse volunteers, but for everyone. Climate change has increased the risks to humans from exposure to ultraviolet light, which impacts health in many ways. Common skin problems include melanoma, basal cell and squamous cell skin cancers, and chronic sun damage. Eyes can be affected by pterygium, cancers of the cornea and conjunctiva, acute solar retinopathy, uveal melanoma, photokeratitis and photoconjunctivitis, and cataracts. Ultraviolet radiation can also negatively affect the immune system. The best way to avoid damage from the sun is to use the following sun safety strategies.

- Avoid direct sun exposure as much as possible during peak UV radiation hours at midday.

- Wear wide-brimmed hats, protective long-sleeved shirts, and long pants.

- Apply sunscreen with a sun protection factor (SPF) of 30 or greater at least 30 minutes before sun exposure and then every few hours thereafter.

- Select contact lenses that offer UV protection.

- Wear sunglasses with high or total UV protection.

SELF-TREATMENT OF TRAVELER'S DIARRHEA

Diarrhea is the most common medical issue amongst travelers to less-developed countries. Traveler's diarrhea is not a specific condition, but is a set of symptoms indicative of an intestinal infection caused by certain bacteria, viruses, or parasites that are transmitted through contaminated food or water. The severity and duration of symptoms depend upon which micro-organism is causing the illness.

Three main types of diarrhea exist, classified by symptoms—watery diarrhea, bloody diarrhea, and chronic diarrhea.

- More than half of travelers have watery diarrhea caused by a toxin-producing bacteria. The symptoms range from several loose, watery stools per day to a more profound illness with profuse diarrhea accompanied by nausea, vomiting, abdominal cramps, and low-grade fever. Symptoms usually last 3–5 days, and dehydration is the main concern.

- Some travelers have bloody diarrhea. This type results from a more serious intestinal infection that invades and inflames the intestinal wall. Symptoms include bloody diarrhea, fever, and abdominal pain. Antibiotics should be started, and sufficient fluids are needed to prevent dehydration.

- A small number of travelers develop chronic diarrhea, and it is usually caused by Giardia. Symptoms include vague abdominal pain, bloating, nausea, anorexia, fatigue, weight loss, and low-grade fever. Treatment is usually a course of metronidazole or tinidazole.

Prevention includes following strict food and water safety guidelines and performing good hand washing.

Most incidents of diarrhea are caused by bacteria sensitive to the quinolone antibiotics. Therefore, you need to have an antibiotic purchased prior to departure with you during your assignment. If bacteria cause a gastrointestinal illness, it is not advisable to take medications such as Pepto-Bismol or Imodium that would contain the organisms in the GI tract, rather than expelling them. Consequently, most travelers take along a course of Cipro or whatever the provider at the travel medicine clinic prescribes, and if they become ill with severe diarrhea, they self-treat with both antibiotic and Pepto-Bismol. Treatment can turn a 3- to 4-day illness into a 1-day illness. Antibiotic resistance exists around the world, so your travel health provider can give you the appropriate prescription for your destination. You also need to discuss with your primary care provider safety issues concerning antibiotics that are related to age, pregnancy, and allergies. Replacement of lost fluids and electrolytes is still the core of treatment. Bringing along oral rehydration salts in your medical kit is important. Avoid stomach irritants, such as coffee, alcohol, and spicy and greasy foods until you are totally well. Imodium is sometimes used to manage the symptoms but should be taken with an antibiotic to avoid retention of possible bacteria that can cause constipation and bloating.

DENTAL EMERGENCIES

Dental problems are very common and rank second to traveler's diarrhea as a medical issue that might arise when you are on a mission. A thorough dental exam prior to departure is very important. Dental pain originates either from inflammation of the dental pulp or from periodontitis, originating around the bone and ligament of the root apex. Local anesthetics and anti-inflammatory medication help. Oral infections can often progress to a full-blown abscess, which is usually accompanied by swelling and pain. Incision and drainage is the treatment of choice, if it can be managed in a remote environment.

Trauma or fracture of the teeth can occur, causing pain and thermal sensitivity. Those engaged in contact sports or sports with a risk of facial injury should wear mouthguards. More severe trauma could result in broken facial bones that would require evacuation and specialized medical attention. Any sharp edges on the broken tooth should be smoothed over with a file or covered with wax. Cavit is a temporary filling material that requires no mixing and is easy to use. It is a good choice to relieve pain and thermal sensitivity. Good oral care and regular dental exams are a must to avoid dental problems, especially in the months prior to departure. Your medical kit should include essential dental items. In the sidebar below, Gary Arnet, DDS, offers advice for emergencies.

DENTAL EMERGENCIES

Treatment of a toothache consists of locating the painful tooth and checking for any obvious cavity or fracture. Clean out any food with a toothbrush, toothpick, or similar tool. Then soak a small cotton pellet or a small piece of cloth in a topical anesthetic, such as a eugenol or benzocaine solution. This should then be placed in the cavity. A small pair of dental tweezers, like the type provided in commercial toothache kits, tick-removing tweezers, or a small instrument such as a toothpick is helpful in placing the cotton, as it is often hard to get your fingers into the mouth. This topical anesthetic should give quick relief. The type of topical anesthetic used is important. Dentists use pure eugenol for emergency treatment of toothaches since it is long-lasting, but this can be difficult to find. Oil of cloves is the same thing and is available without prescription at pharmacies and some health food stores. Be careful, however, as pure oil of cloves can cause chemical burns to the mouth and tongue if it gets off the tooth. Commercial toothache medications that are available include Red Cross Toothache Medicine, containing 85% eugenol, Dent's Toothache Drops, containing benzocaine and eugenol, and Orajel, containing benzocaine. Some products include the small dental tweezers and cotton pellets that you will need. Once the medicated cotton is in place, cover it with a temporary filling material such as Tempanol or Cavit to prevent it from falling out. These are all soft, putty-like materials that can be molded into the cavity. If they are not available, soft dental wax or softened wax from a candle can be used. If a candle is used, melt some wax and let it cool until it is pliable before placing in the mouth.

A pain medication such as 800mg Motrin can be taken every 8 hours. Do not place aspirin on the gum next to a painful tooth. It doesn't help, and it causes a large, painful burn to the gum tissue. (Arnet, 2011).

Only once in all of Rhonda's travels did she need to abort a trip because of a medical problem, and it was a dental emergency. In the northern hill country of Burma (Myanmar), a tooth broke and exposed a nerve. At that time she was not carrying any dental supplies, such as Cavit, in her medical kit. It was a harrowing 2 days as she tried to organize flights out of this remote area, where nobody spoke English. Finally she got to Bangkok, where she found an excellent dentist who was referred by an MD living in Nepal.

SAFE SEX AND POST-EXPOSURE PROPHYLAXIS

Sexually transmitted infections (STIs) represent a major public health problem, and travelers can be at a higher risk for acquiring an STI. Though the majority of many STIs are transmitted in developing countries, the rates of infection continue to grow in the developed world as well. Global travel and migration are significant contributing factors.

Viral STIs, which have become chronic diseases with the wide usage of antiretroviral medications, and difficult to treat, are also on the increase. Hepatitis B is now recognized as an STI. The most significant viral STI is HIV infection leading to AIDS, which at present is a debilitating and fatal disease for many people worldwide who have no access to HAART management (highly active antiretroviral treatment). Human papillomavirus (HPV) can cause cervical cancer, and genital herpes can produce open sores leading to a significantly higher risk of developing other STIs and HIV. Hepatitis B can produce a long-term carrier state resulting in cirrhosis, cancer, and death.

Almost all STIs share common risk factors and common preventive measures. Risk factors include having sex with multiple partners or sex with someone who has had multiple sex partners; engaging in unsafe sexual practices with a homosexual partner; having unprotected sex with anyone who is infected; having sex with prostitutes and drug users; being a long-term expatriate; and being a long-distance truck driver. Additional risk factors exist for viral blood-borne pathogens, along with accompanying additional measures for their prevention.

Preventive measures include abstinence, having mutually monogamous sex with an uninfected partner, or using condoms all the time when otherwise sexually active. Using a diaphragm with spermicidal jelly has also been demonstrated to help reduce risk. Note that condom and diaphragm use can only reduce risk; they don't eliminate it completely.

Those on a short- or long-term volunteer mission have a unique set of circumstances that puts them at additional risk for acquiring an STI while away from home. Volunteers are away from family and societal constraints on behavior. Alcohol use might be increased, thus lowering inhibitions and judgment. Volunteers can be faced with more temptations and opportunities for sexual relationships than at home. Condoms might not be sold abroad or might be of poor quality. Potential partners often hide their past drug and sexual histories, deceiving unwary travelers. And international travel for volunteers from countries with lower prevalence rates can often mean going to other countries where these diseases are much more prevalent than at home.

As a health care provider, you are at a higher risk of contracting HIV because of an accidental needlestick, a cut with a sharp object, or contact of your mucous membranes and non-intact skin with an infected patient's blood or body fluids.

Post-exposure prophylaxis (PEP) with antiretroviral medications decreases the risk of seroconversion by approximately

81%. In areas of sub-Saharan Africa where seroprevalence in certain cities can be more than 25%, any exposure warrants PEP treatment. You should bring a 2-week supply of PEP medications for use in the event of an exposure and begin taking them right away if exposed. Then seek medical attention from a knowledgeable professional and obtain a sample of blood from the source patient if possible. Your prescribing doctor can go over the medications and how to take them.

Hepatitis C is also a blood-borne risk, but no vaccination or PEP is available.

SAFETY AND LEGAL ISSUES

Safety is a concern whether you volunteer in your own community or abroad. The safety measures you take with money and on the street apply both in your own city or town and in distant settings. However, you are likely to feel more vulnerable to a host of problems when far from home and family. In many instances, you really are more vulnerable to such problems as crime, exposure to illicit drugs and sex, and certain legal and cultural issues unique to the country where you are traveling or working. Unless you educate yourself ahead of time about the people, values, religion, and traditions of the region where the mission is going to take place, you run the risk of making mistakes in a variety of areas. Assuming that others share your values, culture, and legal traditions can lead to much unnecessary anguish.

While we covered safety in Chapter 7, it bears some repeating. Safety on the street requires the same common sense that you would exercise at home. Always get good directions from a reliable source before you venture out. Avoid crowded, unfamiliar places such as buses, shared taxis, marketplaces, and marginal areas of a community whenever possible. Be wary of scams. Be aware of your surroundings. You are less likely to be the target of scam artists if you look purposeful as you travel about. Things that seem too good to be true—like ridiculously low prices—probably are and might be a come-on to lure you elsewhere. When lost, seek out people in authority, such as policemen or bank guards. If you have a cell phone that works, have important numbers on speed dial for emergencies.

Protect your money and passport at all times. You should carry a minimal amount of money on your person, and it should not be placed where pickpockets have access to rob you. We recommend that you use a hidden wallet to keep your passport and other items at all times. In addition, avoid opening this wallet in front of others, because this might put you at risk. Most volunteer sites have somewhere that you can lock your valuables. If you bring along other valuables, such as a camera or laptop computer, make sure that you also have a secure place to store them. If you cannot ensure their safety, then it is best to leave them at home. Many volunteer settings have access to a computer or Internet service on-site or at Internet cafes. Finally, it is really best to wear minimal or no jewelry while traveling. Expensive items not only serve to put you at personal risk, but also advertise wealth to the local people.

You also must learn about the legal issues of your host country. Generally, the sponsoring organization can ensure that you are informed about essential issues, but as volunteers you cannot assume to know the laws and customs in the host setting.

RESPECT FOR THE HOST SETTING ENVIRONMENT

Many volunteers find the local environment unsettling at first, with the lack of accustomed modern infrastructures. Unpaved roads, trash along roadways, and lack of the infrastructure common in most developed countries can give the new volunteer the impression that the people lack concern for their environment. This is not the case. We see many examples of those who sweep the dirt around their homes and make efforts to beautify their living environments. The challenges for the environment emerge when governments lack the capacity for trash collection and disposal. Further, families have little ability to dispose of trash other than burning it.

You must ensure that your actions are respectful to the local population and their environment in personal and professional practice. We encourage the use of reusable tote bags, making sure that food is served in reusable plates and that beverages are in recyclable glass bottles. Additionally, consider the appropriate use of plastic in your professional practice and the safe disposal of any hazardous waste. Health Care Without Harm (2011) works to advance healthy communities globally, and current projects concern the safe elimination of mercury and medical waste disposal globally. In Chapter 1 we discussed the importance of healthy environments, carcinogen exposure from the burning of plastics and other refuse, and hazardous environmental exposures from improper pharmaceutical waste, and offered resources for nurses. We must all practice according to the standards of practice in our own home country. The American Nurses Association (2010) recently released the second edition of *Scope and Standards of Nursing Practice*. Standard 16 requires that nurses practice in an environmentally safe and healthy environment. Further, the standards require that nurses participate in strategies to promote healthy environments. As nurse volunteers, we must educate ourselves to be personally and professionally responsible for the host setting environment, remembering that we are guests and must respect the local environment.

LARGER IMPLICATIONS OF OUR WORK

If this is your first time serving in disaster relief or in a distant or international setting, you are likely to find each day full of new experiences and challenges. At the same time, you are also likely to reflect and evaluate your work and think ahead to possible improvements or ways you hope to build upon the work you have begun with your host partners.

THE BENEFITS FOR THE VOLUNTEER

Volunteering is the act of sharing your time, your energy, and your expertise with others, but it is at the same time a "selfish" way to feel good about yourself. Almost to a person, volunteers return from assignments feeling that they have learned much more than they have given. They know more about themselves, and they have had the added opportunity to be immersed in another culture. This is probably the result of working with people whom they would otherwise never meet and gaining an appreciation of how well-off they are in their own country. Pamela Llewellyn writes, "The VSO logo reads 'Sharing Skills, Changing Lives.' Most people volunteering to work in a developing country go hoping to give something of themselves for the benefit of others. They may not fully appreciate how their own lives will be irrevocably changed, too. Sharing skills may change the lives of ordinary and professional people in a volunteer's host country, but the challenge is enormous. Sharing skills will definitely change the volunteer's life" (Pamela Llewellyn, personal communication, 2010).

We devote more discussion to this topic in our final chapter, but urge you as a volunteer to take time to reflect upon all you are receiving from the experience while you are there. Taking time each day or two to capture your thoughts in a journal can help you process not only the intensity of your immersion experience but also can help you after you depart. The final sidebar in this chapter is contributed by Evelyn Gaudrault, MA, RN, the founder of Intercultural Nursing, Inc.

CHANGING LIVES

BUILDING AN ORGANIZATION

Evelyn Gaudrault, MA, RN, served as a nurse in the Peace Corps in Tunisia, North Africa, and noted that many nurses wanted to be able to have a Peace Corps experience but could not do so because of their personal lives. She had a dream to provide short-term volunteer experiences for nurses for learning and service as she had experienced in the Peace Corps. In 1985, while in her master's program in international studies, she collaborated with a faculty member to begin a service project in Haiti that became the organization Intercultural Nursing, Inc. (INI). Applying knowledge learned in a leadership course, an evaluation course, and her thesis, she was able to develop a program that has been sustained for almost 27 years. Local friends helped her establish nonprofit status, a nurse educator helped establish continuing education credits through the

Massachusetts Nurses Association, another friend designed the logo, and others helped to recruit the initial volunteers. INI is a nonprofit, charitable organization that offers nurses, other health care professionals, and nonmedical volunteers an opportunity to work in Haiti or the Dominican Republic. INI participants made three trips yearly to serve in four communities in the Dominican Republic and also in Port au Prince, Haiti. Since that time, hundreds of nurses have participated, many returning year after year.

Though Evelyn turned over the leadership to others after 9 years as the president, the program continues to serve the rural poor in the Dominican Republic and the urban poor in Haiti. The goals of INI are to "provide a consciousness-raising experience for participants looking at third-world realities and the realities of the U.S., to offer a cross cultural education experience for nurses, and to provide health care for the poor and education in the spirit of true exchange." Evelyn notes that INI continues to be blessed by God and the goodness of many people who chose to volunteer and to keep the organization viable for so many years. She notes, "We will always be indebted to the beautiful, warm, and loving people of Haiti and the Dominican Republic who welcomed us into their countries. They touched our hearts and in many instances have changed our lives" (Evelyn Gaudrault, personal communication, 2011).

After hearing the words of many of the volunteers, she states that for many, their hearts were touched and their lives changed. Professionally, they saw how culture impacts health, illness, and treatment. They learned about tropical diseases, poverty, and malnutrition. Once home, they applied their new knowledge to patients from diverse backgrounds. On a personal level, many participants spoke of how they changed their attitudes, perceptions, and worldviews. Some made changes in how they spent their time and money and focused less on staying busy *and more on spending quality time with family and friends. In addition, many volunteers expressed that the experience had a profound spiritual impact upon them.*

More than 75 people attended the 25th anniversary celebration of INI in June 2009 in Topsfield, Massachusetts, USA, with some attendees traveling east from as far away as Washington State and Arizona. The impact of the INI experience was evident among the participants. Many continue to serve with INI, but almost every nurse volunteer in attendance had gone on to serve with Doctors Without Borders, Health Volunteers Overseas, or other global health volunteer organization. Others had created service programs in their community (Evelyn Gaudrault, personal communication, 2011).

When Evelyn dreamed of offering short-term volunteer opportunities for nurses to serve cross-culturally, she not only began an organization that has served the poor in Haiti and the Dominican Republic for the past 27 years, but she also launched a growing group of volunteers who have extended the goals of INI well beyond the borders of the two countries. Indeed, she has touched lives across the world through her dream and hard work. Thank you, Evelyn, from all the nurses who have followed your dream.

BECOMING AN EFFECTIVE VOLUNTEER

- Plan for the time and logistics of your arrival in the volunteer setting.
- Take time to settle into the new environment.
- Recognize that you are likely to experience "culture shock" in the early days of your assignment.

- Be respectful of the host culture always and everywhere.
- Learn to work collaboratively with volunteer team and host partners.
- Allow time for rest, relaxation and rejuvenation.
- Examine your expectations and consider preconceived attitudes of your own and your hosts.
- Learn from our nurses who share their stories in our "Changing Lives" sections.
- Plan for safe food and water.
- Take precautions for insect and animal bites.
- Be mindful of sun safety.
- Learn how to prevent and manage traveler's diarrhea.
- Learn how to care for dental emergencies when you cannot access dental care.
- Practice safe sex and consider post-exposure prophylaxis.
- Consider safety and legal issues in the volunteer setting.
- Respect the host setting environment.
- Consider the implications of volunteer work for building a better future and for the personal impact upon your life.

CHAPTER 9

COMING HOME AND
MOVING FORWARD

In this chapter, we discuss two important issues. First, we consider issues that you will face with the termination of the volunteer assignment, whether at home or abroad. In particular we speak to the adjustments that nurses make when they have been living in a volunteer setting very different from their home setting. Second, we address how nurses can move forward to make contributions to the volunteer setting after they arrive home.

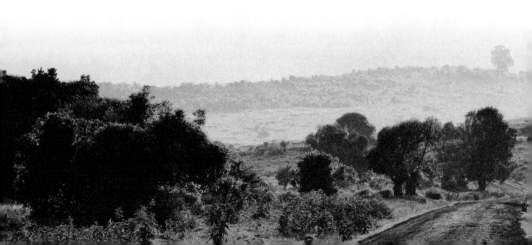

COMPLETING YOUR VOLUNTEER EXPERIENCE

Nurses who volunteer in local settings might continue their commitment for decades, as Diane Martins has in her work with homeless people (see sidebar in Chapter 1). Other volunteers have traveled to locations within their own country or abroad. The completion of their work includes departure to return home. For those of you who are completing your work as a volunteer in a local setting, we do offer suggestions in this chapter that can help you with the termination phase of your work. Though you do not travel, you still likely experience some of the adjustments we discuss in this chapter.

For any volunteer, preparing for departure from the volunteer setting is important. As with any relationship in nursing, you must begin termination long before you actually depart. Throughout the weeks or months you are serving, you should offer regular reminders to your partners about the length of time you are volunteering. As your departure date gets closer, you need to consider allowing time for good-bye visits and opportunities to thank your partners for the opportunity to work with them. In some situations, it is culturally appropriate to give or receive gifts from those you work with. After working a couple of months with nurses in Uganda, Jeanne made a point of taking each of the nurses she worked closely with out to eat in one of the local Kampala restaurants. Likewise, you must learn about the culture of gift giving and receiving in various cultures; specifically, learn when it would be rude to not accept a gift, even if the giver has little to give and you perceive the gift to be too much. Many nurses travel home with lighter luggage, because they leave clothing and donate supplies to people in the community. Jeanne has donated most of the clothes and shoes she brings, unused supplies and packaged food items, flashlights, and stethoscopes and sphygmomanometers. We urge you to consider where to donate these items. Review our comments in Chapter 7 about appropriate donations. These items can be replaced at home but are often treasured by the people where she has volunteered.

If you have served in a poorer country, you need to realize that many of those you have worked with are not free to depart their challenging surroundings, whereas you as a volunteer can return to the comforts of your own home. Additionally, some of the host partners must make adjustments each time a volunteer team departs. Program coordinators have told us that they experience the cycle of sadness that the local hosts feel with each departing team. Be respectful that your departure causes pain for your partners as well as for you. Depending upon the length of time you have been volunteering, the type of setting, and the friends you have made, expect to have sad feelings yourself as you leave. Many of us have been fortunate enough to return to the same location regularly and renew friendships with local people, but even so, you might feel sad in anticipation of your departure and for weeks at home after you return. Unfortunately, Jeanne had a difficult departure day from one of her volunteer trips to Uganda. The morning she left, she had worked with Ugandan nursing students in the hospital on a pediatric unit where two of the babies were dying from malaria. It was difficult enough to leave the many friends she had made during her stay, but the sadness of seeing yet more children suffer from malaria, HIV, and other serious illnesses made her trip home very emotional. For those who have served in disaster or war-time settings, the emotional burden is even greater. In Chapter 5, we discussed that all disaster response must include mental health services for those affected by the disaster (Plum & Veenema, 2003) but also must consider the effects upon nurses who work in disasters as well (Plum, 2003). Volunteers inevitably are affected by the tragedy they witness in the disruption, violence, displacement, and suffering of the victims of disasters (Hewison, 2003; Selby, Jones, Clark, Burgess, & Beilby, 2005).

READJUSTING TO LIFE BACK HOME

Returning home at the completion of your assignment is going to require adjustments on your part. The experiences you have had, the people who have helped you, the friends you have made, and the ones you have helped often have a profound effect on you. Depending on the length of time you were away, you might feel that too many things have changed. Changes in your home or work life might have occurred since you left. Many nurse volunteers use vacation time for their volunteer service, and faculty often plan student immersion trips during breaks in academic schedules. This timing means that nurses and nursing students often must return immediately to the workplace or school with very limited time to process the experience. The abrupt move from the daily routine in a volunteer setting, however busy and exhausting the work might have been, to the fast pace of most work environments today can exact a physical and emotional toll on the nurse volunteer. We recommend that you try to include a few days off between your return from being on assignment in a volunteer setting and your return to work in the home setting.

Physically, nurse volunteers can experience fatigue and residual effects to the gastrointestinal system from the changes in food or water even if no food- or water-borne pathogen is present. In addition, some volunteers might have contracted an infection that must be treated upon return home. Any fever or infection that develops within 2–3 weeks of your return should be checked by your primary care provider. You need to report where you have traveled as well.

However, the physical adjustments are usually minimal and not as challenging as the emotional adjustments. Just as you might have experienced culture shock when you arrived at your assigned site, you might now have reverse culture shock. By that, we mean that you have lived in another culture and return to your home setting seeing things through a new lens. Many sites where volunteers serve are in developing countries. For nurse volunteers who live in countries with higher economic wealth, the disparities can be striking. Supplies are many times in short supply or unavailable. Technology that we take for granted might be nonexistent. You might be overwhelmed by the largesse that we experience in the developed world. The amount of disposable materials that we consume might be disturbing to you when you remember how in the developing world, your colleagues make do with so little. Some returning nurses share their feelings about the focus upon clothing, personal items, cosmetics, and entertainment in their home setting. The large shopping malls, the supermarkets, and the opportunities for consumption at home overwhelm others. Even the ease of getting back into an automobile and traveling on well-maintained roads causes nurse volunteers to view their own home culture with the sense that it is new and uncomfortable. Others comment upon the luxury of hot showers and indoor plumbing that remind them daily of how their global partners live with so much less. Pamela Llewellyn of the United Kingdom states,

> Before I left the U.K. for my VSO placement in Uganda, I met a young teacher who had just returned from Zambia. She said that the going and the staying were easy compared to the difficulties of coming home. Since then I have heard many returned volunteers express similar sentiments. Having returned myself, I too am experiencing those difficulties. At the same time you are missing people and positive experiences in the placement country, you struggle with things about your home country. Supermarkets, consumerism, television, wasted food, Christmas, complaints about public services, and self-indulgence are just a few situations that I am not living easily with. Volunteering is a life-changing experience, in more ways than you would expect (Pamela Llewellyn, personal communication, 2010).

It is very natural to be sad about leaving your colleagues that you worked with and friends that you made during your assignment. Acknowledge your feelings, and do not hesitate to seek counseling if these feelings of loss or frustration are more that you can deal with alone. The organization that you served with might offer this help. Talking with past volunteers and sharing your trip report with them might also help you realize the emotions you are dealing with are normal.

Additionally, you might experience the feeling that you could have done more during your time away. You are likely to be very busy and feel that you are making a difference during your volunteer experience. However, upon your return home you might question how much of a difference you have actually made in the lives of those who suffer greatly and have so little. These feelings are normal and can help you to process your experience and learn how to work toward creating better health for people worldwide. Carol Etherington, a 30-year volunteer in war-torn countries, writes, "To the many back home who asked 'why did you go?'...because nursing in war zones challenges every skill, belief, and value that I have and because nurses bring a dimension of care to suffering people like no other professionals" (Etherington, 1995). We believe that nurses do make a difference; otherwise we would not continue our work, nor would we encourage you to volunteer!

Clare Lawrance, a contributor to this book, offered the following tips to use on your return home.

- Family and friends will be excited to have you back and want to know what it was like or how it feels to be back. Telling them will be difficult, because you won't be able to condense everything into just one conversation, and you might not know what you feel like yet!

- Expect to feel some reverse culture shock. Supermarkets might feel overwhelming, the price of things will astound you, and waste will horrify you.

- Give yourself time to adjust to missing the friends and colleagues you have just left behind. Make sure you have a way to communicate before you leave if you want to be able to stay in touch.

- Attend a debriefing session with your volunteering organization if available—it's good to hear other people's experiences and put yours in perspective.

RECOGNIZING THE BENEFITS OF THE EXPERIENCE

Though you might return home with positive feelings and the energy that result from knowing that you gave your best to help others, you might need time to fully process what you have gained from the experience. Earlier in this book, we recommended that you write a journal during your volunteer experience for reflection and to help to process your feelings. You might have been unable to do so while busy in your volunteer setting, but we urge you to begin or to continue one upon your return home. In this way you can identify the personal impact of the experience. Much of what is written about the positive effects of nurse volunteering comes from the responses of our nurse colleagues. They note that not only did they learn about other cultures and how culture impacts health and illness, and learn to appreciate the work of the host partners to address health concerns, but also that their experiences improved their clinical assessment skills, their ability to work with interdisciplinary teams, and their understanding of the implications of culture upon health and illness (Callister & Cox, 2006; Kollar & Ailinger, 2002; Sloand, Bower, & Groves, 2008).

JoAnn Sampson, RN, who made four volunteer trips to the Dominican Republic writes,

> When I reflect back on my experience in the Dominican Republic, I remember we would often get a bit discouraged knowing that soon we would disappear from these people's lives and take our clinics and our medicines with us. However, just knowing that our presence was there, touching each person with compassion and love and allowing ourselves to receive their unbridled love and spirit became a mutual healing for us all. We were all the healers and the healed! It was a mutual gift, the best medicine of all, with lingering pleasant side effects, no expiration dates, and refills as able (JoAnn Sampson, personal communication, 2011).

One of our contributors describes her feelings about her volunteer experience over a period of 6 years and shows us how reflection helps us to grow over time. She explains that volunteering has phases of adjustment just like the processes of growing up and grieving. During her first year as a volunteer, she was so excited and positive, because she thought she could make everyone happy and fix everything. Then in the second and third years, she became increasingly frustrated that she could not change the world, eliminate poverty, and provide the health care that everyone needed. In her fourth year, she came to the realization that it is all about doing the best you can do in each situation, respecting local knowledge, and sharing your knowledge and skills with your colleagues at every opportunity. She came to know that this was the lasting effect of her efforts as a volunteer. Now her goal is to address the larger issues that create health inequality worldwide and to work with programs that improve sustainability through partnerships. The acceptance of this reality gave her the motivation to continue her work. She also reflects that she continues to question her motivation, because she hopes that her continued interest is not a selfish one, and because she believes that she gains more from the experience than she is able to give to others.

SHARING YOUR EXPERIENCE WITH OTHERS

Friends, colleagues, and family will ask you about your experience. They probably do not want all the details, just the highlights. For some people, knowing that you survived the experience intact is enough. Some nurses who are thinking of volunteering might be interested more in the living conditions and hearing about the nursing services that you provided. Try to elicit from the person who is asking you about the experience what parts they are interested in, so that you can tailor your response.

You can share your experiences in many ways. Offer to talk to prospective volunteers about your experiences, as it can help you to organize your thoughts about them and give you a chance to show what you did. Health Volunteers Overseas (HVO) requires that every volunteer write a trip report that is published on the HVO website. Prospective volunteers can contact the previous volunteers to learn more about the program and the possible match for their needs. It provides you, as the returning volunteer, the opportunity to voice your feelings and reflect upon your experiences. If any groups such as service clubs, your institution or hospital, or your family helped to finance your trip or donated supplies, you need to offer to do a presentation for them. Again it is most important to consider how your presentation portrays the host community. Careful review of presentation content and discussion must reflect respect for the culture and the host community (Center for Global Health, 2009). The impact of this presentation frequently can increase the willingness of the donors to sustain their participation in efforts to help. Writing short newspaper items and offering to speak on local radio programs about your experience are also ways to stimulate interest in your community.

Jeanne and Julia have both given many presentations to church and civic groups that help raise awareness of global health needs and ways that people can be of help without leaving home. In addition, nursing students who have traveled with faculty members usually present their experiences to campus and community groups upon their return in order to further advance knowledge and engage other volunteers.

MOVING FORWARD

The impact of your volunteer experience can be a catalyst for important service to others even when you are back in your home environment. This not only serves to help the volunteer reconcile the disparities between home and volunteer setting, but also helps our profession make lasting impacts upon the health of people worldwide. We do this by helping to build sustainable programs and by continuing the work at home.

BUILDING PROGRAMS

Increasingly, the nursing literature speaks to the importance of sustainability and sustainable partnerships (Leffers & Mitchell, 2011; Memmott et al., 2010; Powell, Gilliss, Hewitt, & Flint, 2010). Sustainable change must be built upon a long-term commitment to system reform by capacity building in the host setting. Relationships that involve reciprocity and equal benefits to both the volunteers and the host partners are essential for service learning but also for service partnerships between volunteer organizations and those served. Memmott et al. (2010) identify key factors in the establishment of sustainable international experiences in an educational program that include finding a fit with the mission of the academic partners and hosts, selecting an appropriate model for study or service, selecting and developing faculty, developing the site, selecting the students, and designing the course. These factors can be translated into factors for volunteer programs as well. The fit we discussed in Chapter 4 ensures that the volunteers sustain the mission of the volunteer partnership. Selection of appropriate volunteers advances the partnership and program success, and designing the program collaboratively advances the partnership to build the capacity of the host partners.

Partnerships that are built at the request of host partners offer the greatest potential for serving the needs of the hosts. Though this is not always possible, sometimes it leads to great success, as with this example of how the first HVO nursing education program was built. Speciosa Mbabali, the first chairperson of the Makerere University, Department of Nursing, initiated the first HVO nursing education program in 2001 in Uganda. Recognizing the need for capacity building as Makerere University began the first BSN program, she sought the help of nurses from the United States. Through the HVO Uganda coordinator, Josephine Buruchara, Speciosa contacted Julia Plotnick and Marie O'Toole to develop a partnership between U.S. nurse volunteers from HVO and the faculty at Makerere University. The initial goal was to strengthen pediatric programs to address the high infant and child mortality rates in Uganda. Early volunteers served for 3–6 months and developed the entire pediatric nursing curriculum for the nursing program. There has been continued service to this partnership, and it has extended into other clinical areas beyond pediatrics. The host partners always help to plan the volunteer assignment, and the volunteer and Makerere faculty members or Mulago Hospital nurses work collaboratively to address the host partner needs. The following sidebar shares some of Speciosa's thoughts on HVO and the partnership.

CHANGING LIVES

The Department of Nursing has played a key role in the official introduction of new HVO arrivals for registration with the Uganda Nurses and Midwives Council and for introduction to Mulago Hospital officials. The department has received HVO nurses both for teaching in the department and for clinical support in Mulago National, the teaching and research hospital. By and large, the teaching has covered courses in pediatrics, physical assessment, health unit administration, curriculum review, and research. In addition, they have provided invaluable guidance and shared experience with faculty. In the hospital, there has been immense support in clinical pediatric nursing.

The HVO volunteers themselves have always expressed happiness at having the opportunity to work in a considerably under-resourced health care environment. This is what has made their work so useful, as they have brought some innovative ideas and experiences to the field.

During the past 10 years, there has been a flow of extremely useful input by different nurse volunteers. To them we owe endless gratitude for having come to our aid even at very difficult times.

CHALLENGES

One of the challenges is that sometimes it has been difficult for them to schedule time to participate in the teaching because of the course arrangements in the semesters, although the department has always found some other equally important assignment to give them.

It is difficult to get volunteers during a global economic recession.

THE FUTURE

We are looking forward to continued support with the HVO program; in fact, we are very hopeful that some volunteers will be found and be able to come and support us as we start our first ever MSN (midwifery focus) program for the fall of 2011.

Thank you for giving us the opportunity to make this contribution (Speciosa Mbabali, personal communication, 2011).

While Speciosa Mbabali served in a faculty and administrative role at Makerere University, Elizabeth Ayebare Ombeva, a current nursing faculty member at Makerere University, was a student nurse in the early days of the BSN program's collaborative work with HVO. Elizabeth shares her experience with HVO beginning when she was an undergraduate nursing student and continuing through her faculty role.

CHANGING LIVES

I am Elizabeth Ayebare Ombeva, a specialist paediatric nurse teaching at the Department of Nursing, Makerere University, Uganda. I have had wonderful experiences with Health Volunteers Overseas (HVO) both as a student and teacher at Makerere University. I have now completed my specialization in paediatric nursing in South Africa and have become a paediatric nursing faculty member.

During my training for the Bachelor of Science in nursing in 2002-03, I was taught by Martha Tanicala, an HVO volunteer who was a specialist paediatric nurse. Martha devoted her time during our paediatric nursing course to teach us clinical skills both in class and on the wards, helping the course coordinator to focus on the theoretical content. She ensured that we gained clinical skills in caring for children, and she changed our attitude toward nursing. This was one of my best rotations as a student nurse.

Due to the passion for children and nursing that Martha had, I was inspired to become a clinical instructor for paediatric nursing when I was appointed to teach in the Department of Nursing. I realised the need to undertake specialisation in paediatric nursing in order to better impart clinical skills to our students. Martha developed course materials that we are still using.

In my first few years as a teaching assistant and clinical instructor for paediatric nursing, I again got an opportunity to work with Jeanne Leffers during the paediatric nursing course. In this course, there is need for the clinical instructor to be on the ward with students, and developing strategies to achieve this goal was challenging. Together we were able to create a model for clinical supervision and demonstrate that on the wards. Due to her long time of experience as a nursing faculty member, Jeanne was a real support to us. She brought along some resources in terms of special books, teaching models, and course materials. Together we developed more course materials such as case studies and planning the allocation of the course curriculum. Jeanne was instrumental in curriculum review for the paediatric nursing course content, since she came at the time when the Bachelor of Science in Nursing curriculum was undergoing review. She has continued to support us with information and advice via e-mails as we have kept in touch with her.

I have now completed my specialization in paediatric nursing in South Africa and have become a paediatric nursing faculty member.

The Department of Nursing at Makerere University has benefited from the Health Volunteers Overseas programme by giving the faculty and students the opportunity to interact with specialist nurses from other countries. This gives our students a global perspective of health and nursing care. My appreciation goes to the sponsors and administrators of this programme. Continue the good work (Elizabeth Ayebare Ombeva, personal communication, March 2011).

Though we offer examples for readers in this book, we do not expect that any volunteer can foresee the eventual outcome for sustainability, particularly on a first assignment. We do suggest that all volunteers read our references on sustainable partnerships (Leffers & Mitchell, 2011; Memmott et al., 2010; Powell, Gilliss, Hewitt & Flint, 2010) to better understand the elements we believe are essential to building programs rather than perpetuating episodic, nonempowering, short-term solutions to larger health problems. Keeping partnership and sustainability as long-term goals will guide nurses as they begin their volunteer experience. Additionally, keeping these goals at the fore when you return home will serve to improve health worldwide.

We offer the example of Ellen Milan, RNC, in the sidebar below as a way to describe how a nurse with particular clinical skills who works side-by-side with her Ugandan nurse partners can achieve impressive and sustained results. Though she might not have been able to foresee the partnership she has built, she began by working collaboratively and seeking to increase the capacity of local nurses to improve their practice. She is an example of a clinical expert whose work with HVO led her to partner with practicing nurses in Uganda to improve the health of at-risk newborns. We also include comments from a Ugandan nurse partner, Damalie Mwogererwa, URM.

CHANGING LIVES

Ellen Milan, RNC, of California first volunteered with Health Volunteers Overseas (HVO) in Uganda in 2001 when she traveled there at the request of Dr. Yvonne Voucher, a California neonatologist. With almost 30 years of clinical experience as a NICU nurse and volunteer experience with Project Concern in San Diego and in Latvia and Romania, she was an ideal candidate to work with the nursing staff at Mulago Hospital to improve the care of newborns. She traveled with Ann Carroll, BSN, NNP, of Maine, for many of her volunteer trips. Together, they worked for 4–6 weeks in the Special Care Babies Unit; taught classes on fetal circulation, stabilization of the neonate, apnea, common respiratory problems, thermoregulation, feeding the high-risk neonate, hypoglycemia, necrotizing enterocolitis, fluid needs, sepsis, and critical assessment techniques for staff; trained them in neonatal resuscitation; and provided teaching materials that they left in the nurses' library after each session. Ellen advises nurse volunteers to come with their teaching materials prepared but to continually revise them to tailor to each particular audience.

Working collaboratively with Ugandan pediatrician Dr. Sarah Nakakeeto, Ellen taught nursing, midwifery, and neonatal resuscitation and thermoregulation. With careful collaboration with the hospital staff, they collected donations appropriate for the setting there (syringe pumps, IV tubing, monitoring electrodes, suctioning devices, resuscitation bags, nasal cannulas, feeding tubes, and stethoscopes) as well as clothing, blankets, and booties for the infants. Ellen even brings a camera and small photo printer. If a mother would like a photo of her baby, Ellen takes a photo, prints it at the guest house, and gives it immediately to the family. These photos are treasures to the mothers and the staff.

Beginning in 2004, Dr. Nakakeeto and neonatologist Dr. Voucher from the United States began to travel to other parts of the country to assess the possibility of creating NICUs in more remote settings. Since that time, Ellen continues to travel throughout the country teaching nurses important skills for high-risk newborn care. With Dr. Nakakeeto and nurses from the Special Care Babies Unit (SCBU) at Mulago, they have been working with the Saving Newborn Lives program and have provided important educational materials and outreach throughout the country. Ellen has been at work building the capacity of the Ugandan nurses as well as building sustainability for neonatal nurse education in Uganda. At the time of writing, two new volunteer U.S. nurses are working with Ellen and Ann Carroll with the goal of building an ongoing program. Ellen's goals for the new team members is to identify specific system-level needs for the admission, high-risk delivery, and transfer to the SCBU to work to improve the nursing procedures that will improve infant outcomes (HVO, 2011; Ellen Milan, personal communication, 2011).

WHAT IT MEANS TO PARTNER/WORK WITH VOLUNTEERS

Ellen has worked in partnership with Damalie Mwogererwa, URM, a Ugandan nursing partner for the past 5 years. Damalie offers these words:

"Volunteers have meant a lot to us and me in particular and more so to the Special Care Nursery.

When I first worked in the unit, I had no knowledge of the care of a sick newborn, and I felt as if it was a punishment to put me in the Special Care Nursery. But when the HVO volunteers came with their training and support at work, they gave me knowledge and confidence to work.

I learned the importance of passing on knowledge to students, my colleagues, and nurses in the community.

They also helped equip the unit with machines and supplies, which made work easier and more interesting.

They are dedicated when working, and it gives me a challenge. I wish to copy them, for example, in monitoring babies, responding to the needs of the babies, feeling compassion for the parents and love for the babies, and a lot more.

Health Volunteer Overseas nurses have meant a lot to us, through the knowledge they share and teaching materials (such as handouts, nursing journal articles, and computer presentations on flash drives) they provide so we can train others, the increasing number of babies surviving, and the equipment to use.

Ellen and Ann are the source of the services we give to the babies and colleagues.

Long life, God bless you, and bless the work of your hands. Amen!"

Damalie Mwogererwa, URM
Special Care Baby Unit
Mulago Hospital, Kampala, Uganda

(Damalie Mwogererwa, personal communication, 2011)

THE WORK CONTINUES AT HOME

If your experience as a volunteer was a good one and you believe the mission of the organization that you selected to serve with is worthwhile, you now have a great opportunity to become an ambassador for the organization where you served. All nongovernment organizations are continually seeking funds, supplies, and volunteers so that they can continue their mission of helping others. You might be the catalyst that spurs a church group or service organization to select your group to receive their efforts, whether fundraising, collecting supplies, recruiting volunteers, or other positive activities.

Marie Walters, B/Nurs, senior lecturer in child nursing at the University of Wolverhampton, served as a volunteer in Malawi. As you will see in the following sidebar, the work she began there continues in a variety of ways to help build support for Queen Elizabeth Central Hospital and for the care of children abroad.

CHANGING LIVES

Marie Walters has worked as a nurse educator at the Queen Elizabeth Central Hospital in Blantyre, Malawi, over the past 4 years for a total of 16 months. During her time there, she worked collaboratively with the Malawian nurses, and she concluded that there were unmet needs regarding pain assessment and management in children. Recognizing that cultural expectations, social norms, language, and the broader culture all impact cultural beliefs about pain and the treatment of pain, Marie sought to collaborate with the Malawian nursing staff to assess and manage children's pain. In addition, she learned that nurses' socialization caused them to have beliefs about opiates as "bad" and dangerous. Further, as a result of the social hierarchy of medical care in countries in Africa, parents who might be the best source of information about pain assessment and pain management have been undervalued in the decision-making process (Walters, 2009). In response to this evidence, Marie conducted an assessment of her Malawian nurse colleagues' beliefs about pain assessment and management. Based upon the findings, she developed educational workshops to address the fears, misconceptions, and myths associated with pain management. United Kingdom partners were eager to learn about the problems that the Malawian nurses face, such as safe storage, prescribing protocols, and the access to analgesic medications.

Collaboratively they developed plans for locked cupboards, dispensing guidelines, protocols, and culturally appropriate

translated pain assessment tools (see www.painsourcebook.ca).
The Faces pain scale translated into Chichewa was developed
through this partnership. Back in the UK, Marie continues to
fundraise for the partnership, orientate new nurses to the project,
and work on project organisation within the partnership team.
Personally she is near to completion of her Master's in Public
Health degree and with her dissertation, "An Interpretative
Phenomenological Analysis of Health Professional's Insights
into Paediatric Pain in Sub-Saharan Africa," she hopes to raise
awareness of this much-neglected area of international child
health, something she remains extremely passionate about. The
work in Malawi continues as more nurses from Birmingham
Children's Hospital volunteer in Malawi on a regular basis.
Additionally, a specialist nurse in burn injuries was sent to
Blantyre for 6 months to work on pain management for children
with burns, an area with much suffering and very few nurses to
manage the heavy workload.

Marie Walters' work shows that there are many ways
to serve globally from your home setting. It is not necessary and often not practical to actually volunteer on-site to
contribute to improving the lives of so many. Another way
to expand your horizons is to offer to serve on committees
that exist in most organizations. Jeanne serves as the country
program director for nursing for Health Volunteers Overseas
in Uganda, a position that she has held for several years. Julia
now serves as chairman of the board at HVO. Both of us serve
on the Nursing Education Steering Committee for HVO as
well.

Finally, we are often not aware of how our influence as
nurses can improve the health and well-being of others. As
nurses with experience serving those people most in need of
our care around the globe, we can influence other people who

move on to create outstanding partnerships on their own. Though neither nurse actually suggested the idea to him, both nurses led by the example of their lives in ways that inspired a remarkable young man. Rye Barcott, who is not a nurse, was influenced by two important nurses in his life—his mother, Dr. Donna Schwartz-Barcott, nurse and anthropologist of the University of Rhode Island, who spent a year working in Peru as a young nurse, and the late Tabitha Atieno Festo, of Kibera, Kenya, who with a small donation from Rye that served as seed money went on to begin a small clinic in her Kibera community. As an undergraduate student at the University of North Carolina (UNC), Rye spent time in Kibera, Kenya, and became inspired by the talents of people such as Tabitha who lived there. In 2001, during his senior year at UNC, he began the organization Carolina for Kibera. According to its website, the organization "exists to develop local leaders, catalyze positive change, and alleviate poverty in the Kibera slum of Nairobi" (http://cfk.unc.edu/). The programs and achievements include a new health care clinic named for nurse Tabitha Atieno Festo, as well as youth empowerment programs, educational initiatives, and programs to promote environmental sustainability (Barcott, 2011).

When you sometimes feel that you have not done enough, that so much more remains to do, always remember that you are not alone in your efforts. An army of nurses might be interested in helping others, and you might be the impetus they need to investigate their own ability to help. Margaret Mead once said: "Never doubt that a small group of thoughtful committed people can change the world; indeed, it's the only way it ever has!"

BECOMING AN EFFECTIVE VOLUNTEER

- Consider the end of your volunteer experience to be important for yourself and for those with whom you serve.

- Review guidelines for appropriate donations.

- Incorporate your experience into your life at home.

- Learn about ways to help your adjustment once you end your volunteer service.

- Recognize the benefits of your experience.

- Share your experience with others.

- Continue to support the work of the program where you volunteered.

- Read about partnership and sustainability issues.

- Learn from nurses worldwide who share their expertise in the "Changing Lives" stories.

- Continue the work at home.

REFERENCES

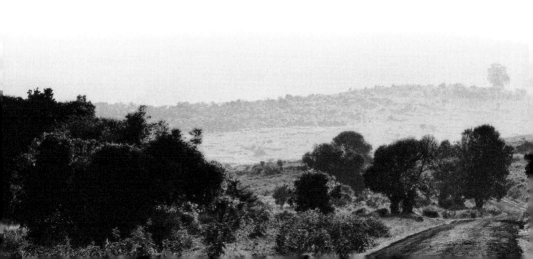

Adams, L. M. (2007). Mental health needs of disaster volunteers: A plea for awareness. *Perspectives in Psychiatric Care,* *43*(1), 52–54.

Ailinger, R. L. (2002). U.S. nursing students in Nicaragua: A community health clinical experience. *Revista Latino-Americana de Enfermagem, 10*(1), 104–105.

Ailinger, R. L., & Carty, R. M. (1996). Teaching community health nursing in Nicaragua. *Nursing and Health Care: Perspective on Community, 17*(5), 236–241.

Ailinger, R. L., Gonzalez, R., & Zamora, L. (2007). Health and illness concepts among lower income Nicaraguan women. *Qualitative Health Research, 17*(3), 382–385.

Ailinger, R. L., Molloy, S., Zamora, L., & Benavides, C. (2000). Nurse practitioner students in Nicaragua. *Clinical Excellence for Nurse Practitioners.* 4(4), 240–244.

Ailinger, R. L., Molloy, S., Zamora, L., & Benavides, C. (2004). Herbal remedies in a Nicaraguan barrio. *Journal of Transcultural Nursing, 15*(4), 278–282.

Allgeyer, K. (2011). The history of nursing with the American Red Cross. Retrieved March 10, 2011, from www.workingnurse.com/articles/The-History-of-Nursing-with-the-American-Red-Cross

Alliance of Nurses for Healthy Environments. (2011). *Safe medication disposal.* Retrieved March 10, 2011, from http://envirn.org/pg/pages/view/4094/safe-medication-disposal

American Association of Colleges of Nursing (AACN). (2008). *The essentials of baccalaureate education for professional nursing practice.* Retrieved March 29, 2011, from www.aacn.nche.edu/Education/essentials.htm

American Nurses Association. (2001). *Code of ethics for nurses.* Retrieved January 6, 2011, from www.nursingworld.org/MainMenuCategories/ThePracticeofProfessionalNursing/EthicsStandards/CodeofEthics.aspx

American Nurses Association. (2005). *Faith community nursing: Scope and standards of practice*. American Nurses Association and Health Ministries Association.

American Nurses Association (ANA). (2010). *Scope and standards of nursing practice* (2nd ed.). Silver Spring, MD: Author.

Anderson, E.T., & McFarlane, J. (2011). *Community as partner: Theory and practice in nursing* (6th ed.). Philadelphia: Lippincott Williams & Wilkins.

Arnet, G. (2011). No dentist? Oh, no! *Backwoods Home Magazine*. Retrieved January 20, 2011, from www.backwoodshome.com/articles2/arnet75b.html

Ball, K. (2003). Deep vein thrombosis and airline travel, the deadly duo. *AORN Journal*. Retrieved January 20, 2011 from http://findarticles.com/p/articles/mi_m0FSL/is_2_77/ai_98134860/

Baran, R. M. (2010). *Global nursing: Fulfilling a dream in Thailand. Reflections on Nursing Leadership, 36* (3). Retrieved April 2, 2011, from www.reflectionsonnursingleadership.org/Pages/Vol36_3_Baran.aspx

Barcott, R. (2011). *It happened on the way to war: A marine's path to peace*. New York: Bloomsbury.

Bennett, C. A. (2001). *Volunteering: The selfish benefits: Achieve deep-down satisfaction and create that desire in others*. Oak View, CA: Committee Communication.

Bertschinger, C., & Blake, F. (2005). *Moving mountains*. London: Doubleday.

Blaustein, A. I. (2003). *Make a difference: America's guide to volunteering and community service*. San Francisco, CA: John Wiley & Sons.

Bosworth, T. L., Haloburdo, E. P., Hetrick, C., Patchett, K., Thompson, M. A., & Welch, M. (2006). International partnership to promote quality care: Faculty groundwork, student projects, and outcomes. *The Journal of Continuing Education in Nursing, 37*(1), 32–38.

Brudenell, I. (2003). Parish nursing: Nursing the body, mind, spirit and community. *Public Health Nursing, 20*(2), 85–94.

Callister, L. C., & Cox, A. H. (2006). Opening our hearts and minds: The meaning of international clinical nursing electives in the personal and professional lives of nurses. *Nursing & Health Sciences, 8*(2), 95–102.

Callister, L. C., & Hobbins-Garbett, D. (2000). Enter to learn, go forth to serve: Service learning in nursing education. *Journal of Professional Nursing, 16*(3), 177–183.

Calvillo, E., Clark, L., Ballantyne, J. E., Pacquiao, D., Purnell, L. D., & Villarruel, A. M. (2009). Cultural competency in baccalaureate nursing education. *Journal of Transcultural Nursing, 20*(2), 137–145.

Campinha-Bacote, J. (2005). A biblically based model of cultural competence in health care delivery. *Journal of Multicultural Nursing and Health, 11*(2), 16–22.

Carter, J. (2008). *A remarkable mother.* New York: Simon and Schuster.

Casey, D., & Murphy, K. (2008). Irish nursing students' experiences of service learning. *Nursing and Health Services, 10*(4), 306–311.

Cavanaugh-Sutkus, S. A. (2008). Service: Improving the health of the world's people: Wisdom from the Brazilian rain forest. *Reflections on Nursing Leadership, 34*(4). Retrieved March 23, 2011, from www.reflectionsonnursingleadership.org/Pages/Vol_34_4_Sutkus.aspx

CBS News. (2010). *Lynn University president says he still believes in miracles.* Retrieved November 30, 2010, from www.cbs12.com/news/media-4723753-university-ross.html

Center for Global Health. (2009). *Towards best practices in the Center for Global Health: Culture shock and communication.* Retrieved April 18, 2011, from http://centerforglobalhealth.wisc.edu/documents/CultureShockandCommunication.pdf

Center for Global Health. (2009). *Towards best practices in the Center for Global Health: First, do no harm—guidelines for donations.* Retrieved April 18, 2011, from http://centerfor-globalhealth.wisc.edu/documents/GuidelinesforDonations.pdf

Central Asia Institute. (2011). Peace and hope begins with education: One child at a time. Retrieved March 10, 2011, from www.ikat.org/projects

Collins, J., DeZerega, S., & Heckscher, Z. (2002). *How to live your dream of volunteering overseas.* New York, NY: Penguin.

Crigger, N., Brannigan, M., & Baird, M. (2006). Compassionate nursing professionals as good citizens of the world. *Advances in Nursing Science, 29*(1), 15–26.

Crigger, N. J. (2008). Towards a viable and just global nursing ethics. *Nursing Ethics, 15*(1), 17–27.

Crigger, N. J., & Holcomb, L. (2007). Practical strategies for providing culturally sensitive, ethical care in developing nations. *Journal of Transcultural Nursing, 18*(1), 70–76.

Crump, J. A., & Sugarman, J. (2008). Ethical considerations for short-term experiences by trainees in global health. *JAMA, 300*(12), 1456–1458.

Crump, J. A., & Sugarman, J. (2010). Global health training: Ethics and best practice guidelines for training experiences in global health. *American Journal of Tropical Medicine & Hygiene, 83*(6), 1178–1182.

Department of Homeland Security. (2011). *National Response Framework.* Retrieved January 6, 2011, from www.fema.gov/emergency/nrf/aboutNRF.htm

Dossey, B. (2010). *Florence Nightingale: Mystic, visionary, healer.* Philadelphia, PA: F. A. Davis.

Duke, J., Connor, M., & McEldowney, R. (2009). Becoming a culturally competent health practitioner in the delivery of culturally safe care: A process oriented approach. *Journal of Cultural Diversity, 16*(2), 40–49.

Emory University. (2010). Nursing students provide health services to migrant farmers in south Georgia. Retrieved November 18, 2010, from http://emoryhealthblog.com/

Etherington, C. (1995). Working in international war zones: A personal account. *Tennessee Nurse, 58*(5), 14–16.

Evanson, T. A., & Zust, B. L. (2006). Bittersweet knowledge: The long term effects of an international experience. *Journal of Nursing Education, 45*(10), 412–419.

Fadiman, A. (1997). *The spirit catches you and you fall down.* New York: Farrar, Straus & Giroux.

Foster, J. (2009). Cultural humility and the importance of long-term relationships in international partnerships. *Journal of Obstetric, Gynecologic and Neonatal Nursing (JOGNN), 38*(1), 100–107.

Fothergill, A., Palumbo, M. V., Rambur, B., Reinier, K., & McIntosh, B. (2005). The volunteer potential of inactive nurses for disaster preparedness. *Public Health Nursing, 22*(5), 414–421.

Fraleigh, J. M. (2010). Crisis nursing in Haiti: One traveler's tale. *Healthcare Traveler,* 34–37. Retrieved from www. healthcaretraveler.com

Gaudrault, E. (1995, Spring). INI newsletter.

Geiger, J. (2010). What we do and why we do it. Keynote address published online by *Doctors for Global Health.* Retrieved April 1, 2011, from www.dgh.online.org/content/faq

Gill, G. (2004). *The Nightingales: The extraordinary upbringing and curious life of Miss Florence Nightingale.* New York: Random House.

Greene, R., & Greene, D. G. (2009). Resilience in the face of disasters: Bridging micro- and macro-perspectives. *Journal of Human Behavior in the Social Environment, 19,* 1010–1024.

Haloburdo, E. P., & Thompson, M. A. (1998). A comparison of international learning experiences for baccalaureate nursing students: Developed and developing countries. *Journal of Nursing Education, 37*(1), 13–21.

Hamner, J. B., Wilder, B., & Byrd, L. (2007). Lessons learned: Integrating service learning community-based partnership into the curriculum. *Nursing Outlook, 55*(2), 106–110.

Health and Human Services. (2011). National Nurse Response Team. Retrieved from www.phe.gov/Preparedness/responders/ndms/teams/Pages/nnrt.aspx

Health Care Without Harm. (2011). Global projects & other regions. Retrieved January 20, 2011, from www.noharm.org/global/

Health Volunteers Overseas (HVO). (2007). *A guide to volunteering overseas* (5th ed.). Retrieved May 2, 2011, from http://www.hvousa.org/pdfs/HVOvolguide2010.pdf

Health Volunteers Overseas (HVO). (2010a). Mission and vision statement. Retrieved October16, 2010, from www.hvousa.org/whoWeAre/mission.shtml

Health Volunteers Overseas (HVO). (2010b). Trip reports. *KnowNET.* Retrieved October 16, 2010, from www.hvousa.org/volunteerToolkit/knownet.shtml

Health Volunteers Overseas (HVO). (2011). Ellen Milan trip reports. Retrieved February 12, 2011, from www.hvousa.org

Herbst, D. (2011). How to volunteer in Haiti. Retrieved January 17, 2010, from www.tonic.com/article/how-to-volunteer-in-haiti/

Heuer, L. J., & Bengiamin, M. I. (2001). American nursing students experience shock during a short-term international program. *Journal of Cultural Diversity, 8*(4), 128–134.

Hewison, C. (2003). Working in a war zone: The impact on humanitarian health workers. *Australian Family Physician, 32*(9), 679–681.

International Council of Nurses (ICN). (2010). *Our mission.* Retrieved November 19, 2010, from www.icn.ch/about-icn/icns-mission/

International Council of Nurses (ICN). (2011). *Disaster planning and relief.* Retrieved from www.icn.ch/publications/disaster-planning-and-relief/disaster-planning-and-relief.html

Institute of Medicine. (2009). *Guidance for establishing crisis standards of care for use in disaster situations.* Retrieved April 4, 2011, from www.iom.edu/Reports/2009/DisasterCareStandards.aspx

International Nursing Coalition for Mass Casualty Education (INCMCE). (2011). Retrieved April 4, 2011, from www.nursing.vanderbilt.edu/incmce/overview.html

Jarrett, S. L., Hummel, F., & Whitney, K. L. (2005). Preparing for the 21st century: Graduate nursing education in Vietnam. *Nursing Education Perspectives, 26*(3), 172–175.

Kingma, M. (2008). Nurse migration and the global health care economy. *Policy, Politics, and Nursing Practice, 9*(4), 328–333.

Kleber, M. (2011). DVT: David Bloom's silent killer. *USA Today.* Retrieved January 20, 2011, from www.usatoday.com/news/health/spotlighthealth/2003-04-11-bloom_x.htm

Kollar, S. J., & Ailinger, R. L. (2002). International clinical experiences: Long term impact on students. *Nurse Educator, 27*(1), 28–31.

Kreutzer, S. (2010). Nursing body and soul in the parish: Lutheran deaconess mother houses in Germany and the United States. *Nursing History Review, 18,* 134–150.

Kuntz, S., Frable, P., Qureshi, K., & Strong, L. (2008). *Disaster preparedness white paper for community/public health nursing educators.* Association of Community Health Nursing Educators. Retrieved from www.achne.org/i4a/pages/index.cfm?pageid=3326

Lange, I., & Ailinger, R. L. (2001). International nursing faculty exchange model: A Chile-USA case. *International Nursing Review*, 48(2), 109–116.

Leffers, J., & Mitchell, E. (2011). Conceptual model for partnership and sustainability in global health. *Public Health Nursing*, 28(1), 91–102.

Legg, T. J. (2009). Nursing in disaster situations: Are you prepared to answer the call? *Pennsylvania Nurse*, 64(2), 4–7.

Levi, A. (2009). The ethics of nursing student international clinical experiences. *JOGNN, 38*(1), 94–99.

Lukasik, C. (1983) International nursing with Project HOPE. *Pediatric Nursing*, 9(4), 267–268.

Lundy, K. S., & Janes, S. (2009). *Community health nursing: Caring for the public's health.* Sudbury, MA: Jones & Bartlett.

Maurer, F. A., & Smith, C. M. (2009). *Community/public health nursing practice: Health for families and populations* (4th ed.). St. Louis, MO: Saunders/Elsevier.

McKinley, J. B. (1994). A case for refocusing upstream: The political economy of illness. In P. Conrad & R. Kern (Eds.), *The Sociology of Health and Illness: Critical Perspectives* (pp. 509–523). New York: St. Martin's Press.

McKinnon, T., & Fealy, G.M. (2011). Core principles for developing global service learning programs in nursing. *Nursing Education Perspectives*, 32(2), 95–101.

Medecins Sans Frontieres, et al. (2010). *Working with humanitarian organisations: A guide for nurses, midwives, and health care professionals.* Retrieved May 2, 2011, from http://www.rcn.org.uk/__data/assets/pdf_file/0007/78757/003156.pdf

Memmott, R. J., Coverston, C. R., Heise, B. A., Williams, M., Maughan E. D., Kohl, J., & Palmer, S. (2010). Practical considerations in establishing sustainable international nursing experiences. *Nursing Education Perspectives*, 31(5), 298–302.

Millennium Development Goals. (2011). *We can end poverty.* Retrieved March 10, 2011, from www.un.org/millennium-goals/bkgd.shtml

Mortenson, G. (2011). A conversation with Greg Mortenson. *Loyola Marymount Magazine.* Retrieved March 3, 2011, from http://magazine.lmu.edu/archive/2010/conversation-greg-mortenson

Mortenson, G. (2009). *Stones into schools: Promoting peace through education in Afghanistan and Pakistan.* New York: Viking Press.

Mortenson, G., & Relin, D. O. (2006). *Three cups of tea: One man's mission to promote peace...one school at a time.* New York: Viking.

Myers, J. (2010). Julie Myers nurse volunteer Uganda. *Doctors for Global Health* blog. Retrieved October 11, 2010, from www.dghonline.org/news/nurse-volunteer-uganda

Narsavage, G. L., Lindell, D., Chen Y. J., Savrin, C., & Duffy, E. (2002). A community engagement initiative: Service-learning in graduate nursing education. *Journal of Nursing Education, 4*(10), 457–461.

Nash, K. (2008). Interprofessional, cross-cultural immersion in Nicaragua. *Reflections on Nursing Leadership, 34*(1). Retrieved March 23, 2011, from www.reflectionsonnursingleadership.org/Pages/Vol34_1_Nash.aspx

Nicholas, P. K., Adejumo, O., Nokes, K., Ncama, B. P., Bhengu, B. R., Elston, E., & Nicholas, T. P. (2009). Fulbright scholar opportunities for global health and women's health care in HIV/AIDS in sub-Saharan Africa. *Applied Nursing Research, 22*(1), 73–77.

Nokes, K. M., Nickitas, D. M., Keida, R., & Neville, S. (2005). Does service-learning increase cultural competency, critical thinking, and civic engagement? *Journal of Nursing Education, 44*(2), 65–70.

Northern volunteer nurses of America's Civil War. (2011). Retrieved March 10, 2011, from www.historynet.com/northern-volunteer-nurses-of-americas-civil-war.htm

Office of Civilian Volunteer Medical Reserve Corps. (2011). *MRC federal deployment competencies.* Retrieved April 4, 2011, from www.medicalreservecorps.gov/file/MRC_ Deployment/MRC-FedDeployComp2.pdf

O'Hara, H. (2006). Public health nursing in Latin America. *Public Health Nursing, 23*(4), 373–375.

O'Neil, E. (2006). *A practical guide to global health service.* Chicago, IL: AMA.

Otterness, N., Gehrke, P., & Sener, I. (2007). Partnerships between nursing education and faith communities: Benefits and challenges. *Journal of Nursing Education, 46*(1), 39–44.

Oxford Dictionaries. (2011). Retrieved January 22, 2011, from http://oxforddictionaries.com/view/entry/m_en_ us1240668#m_en_us1240668

Patsdaughter, C. A., Christensen, M. H., Kelley, B. R., Masters, J. A., & Ndiwane, A. N. (2001). Meeting folks where they are: Collecting data from ethnic groups in the community. *Journal of Cultural Diversity, 8*(4), 122–127.

Peterson, S. J., & Schaffer, M. J. (1999). Service-learning: A strategy to develop group collaboration and research skills. *Journal of Nursing Education, 38*(5), 208–216.

Plum, K. C. (2003). Understanding the psychological impact of disasters. In T. G. Veneema (Ed.), *Disaster nursing and emergency preparedness for chemical, biological, and radiological terrorism and other hazards* (pp. 62–81). New York: Springer.

Plum, K. C., & Veenema, T. G. (2003). Management of psychological effects. In T. G. Veneema (Ed.), *Disaster nursing and emergency preparedness for chemical, biological, and radiological terrorism and other hazards* (pp. 202–221). New York: Springer.

Powell, D. L., Gilliss, C. L., Hewitt, H. H., & Flint, E. P. (2010). Application of a partnership model for transformative and sustainable international development. *Public Health Nursing, 27*(1), 54–70.

Project Hope. (2011). *Delivering health education, medicines, supplies and volunteers where needed.* Retrieved March 23, 2011, from www.projecthope.org/

Pryor, T. (2005). Relationship building and a story of hope in tsunami-ravaged Banda Aceh, Indonesia: Perspective of a US public health service nurse. *American Journal of Critical Care, 14*(6), 474–475.

Qureshi, K., & Veenema, T. G. (2003). Disaster triage and chemical decontamination. In T. G. Veneema (Ed.), *Disaster nursing and emergency preparedness for chemical, biological, and radiological terrorism and other hazards* (pp. 153–170). New York: Springer.

Reliefweb. (2011). *Serving the information needs of the humanitarian relief community.* Retrieved April 4, 2011, from www.reliefweb.int/rw/dbc.nsf/doc100?OpenForm

Riner, M. E., & Becklenberg, A. (2001). Partnering with a sister city organization for an international service-learning experience. *Journal of Transcultural Nursing, 12*(3), 234–240.

Robinson, J. A. (2010). Nursing and disaster preparedness. *International Nursing Review, 57*(2), 148.

Robinson, J. A. (2010). Nursing and health policy perspectives: International collaborative nursing. *International Nursing Review, 57*(4), 405.

Rosenkoetter, M. M. (1997). A framework for international health care consultations. *Nursing Outlook, 45*(4), 182–187.

Rosenkoetter, M. M., & Nardi, D. A. (2007). American Academy of Nursing Expert Panel on Global Nursing and Health: White paper on global nursing and health. *Journal of Transcultural Nursing, 18*(4), 23–34, 305–315.

Royal College of Nursing (RCN). (2010, September). *Working with humanitarian organisations: A guide for nurses, midwives and health professionals.* Retrieved March 24, 2011, from www.rcn.org.uk/__data/assets/pdf_file/0007/78757/003156.pdf

Seifer, S. D. (1998). Service-learning: Community-campus partnerships for health professions education. *Academic Medicine, 73*(3), 273–277.

Selby, S., Jones, A., Clark, S., Burgess, T., & Beilby, J. (2005). Re-entry adjustment of cross cultural workers: The role of the GP. *Australian Family Physician, 34*(10), 863–864, 878.

Shaffer, E. R., Waitzkin, H., Brenner, J., & Jasso-Aguilar, R. (2005). Global trade and public health. *American Journal of Public Health, 95*(1), 23–34.

Sigma Theta Tau International Service Learning Task Force. (2009). Service learning: Pedagogy of civic engagement for nursing. Unpublished manuscript.

Sloand, E., Bower, K., & Groves, S. (2008). Challenges and benefits of international clinical placements in public health nursing. *Nurse Educator, 33*(1), 35–38.

Stanhope, M., & Lancaster, J. (2008). *Public health nursing: Population-centered health care in the community* (7th Ed.). St. Louis: Mosby.

Stokowski, L. (2008). Ready, willing and able: Preparing nurses to respond to disasters. *Medscape.* Retrieved April 4, 2011, from www.medscape.com/viewarticle/579888

Stone, S., & Jones, P. (2008). *Volunteering around the globe: Life-changing travel adventures.* Washington, DC: Capital Books.

Tervalon, M., & Murray-Garcia, J. (1998). Cultural humility versus cultural competence: A critical distinction in defining physician training outcomes in multicultural education. *Journal of Health Care for the Poor and Underserved, 9*(2), 117–125.

The Sphere Project. Retrieved January 22, 2011, from www.sphereproject.org/

Thormar, S., Gersons, B., Juen, B., Marschang, A., Djakababa, M., & Olff, M. (2010). The mental health impact of volunteering in a disaster setting: A review. *The Journal of Nervous and Mental Disease, 198*(8), 529–538.

United Nations High Commission on Refugees. (2011a). UNHCR mission statement. Retrieved January 22, 2011, from www.unhcr.org/pages/49ed83046.html

United Nations High Commission on Refugees. (2011b). Refugees. Retrieved January 22, 2011, from www.unhcr.org/pages/49c3646c125.html

University of Pennsylvania. (2011). *Multicultural/global health care minor.* Retrieved January 20, 2011, from www.nursing.upenn.edu/students.Minors/Pages/MulticulturalGlobalHealthCareMinor.aspx

University of Wisconsin. (2011). *Center for Global Health.* Retrieved April 4, 2011, from www.centerforglobalhealth.wisc.edu

U.S. Department of Health & Human Services. (2009, April 30). 2009—H1N1 flu virus. Retrieved April 18, 2011, from http://www.fda.gov/NewsEvents/Testimony/ucm153570.htm

Veenema, T. G. (2003). Essentials of disaster planning. In T. G. Veneema (Ed.), *Disaster nursing and emergency preparedness for chemical, biological and radiological terrorism, and other hazards* (pp. 3–30). New York: Springer.

Waite, R., & Calamaro, C. J. (2010). Cultural competence: A systemic challenge to nursing education, knowledge exchange, and the knowledge process. *Perspectives in Psychiatric Care, 46*(1), 74–80.

Walters, M. (2009). Pain assessment in sub-Saharan Africa. Pediatric Pain Letter, 11(3), 22–26.

Warner, J. R. (2002). Cultural competence immersion experiences: Public health among the Navajo. *Nurse Educator,* 27(4), 187–190.

Watson, S. M. (2010). *Hidden treasures: Four great reasons to sign up for an international mission. Reflections on Nursing Leadership,* 36(2). Retrieved March 23, 2011, from www.reflectionsonnursingleadership.org/Pages/Vol36_2_Watson.aspx

Werner, D., Thuman, C., & Maxwell, J. (2010). *Where there is no doctor*. Berkeley, CA: Hesperian Foundation.

What role did women play in World War II. (2011). Retrieved March 10, 2011, from www.megaessays.com/viewpaper/8948.html

Wilson, L. L. (2011). The world as community: Globalization and health. In *Community as Partner: Theory and Practice in Nursing* (6th ed.), pp. 2–15. Philadelphia: Wolters Kluwer.

Wood, M. J., & Atkins, M. (2006). Immersion in another culture: One strategy for increasing cultural competency. *Journal of Cultural Diversity, 13*(1), 50–54.

World Health Organization. (2009). *Global standards for the initial education of professional nurses and midwives*. Retrieved May 2, 2011, from http://www.who.int/hrh/nursing_midwifery/en/

World Health Organization (WHO). (2011). *Health action in crises*. Retrieved April 4, 2011, from www.who.int/hac/about/en/

World Health Professions Alliance (WHPA). (2007). *A core competency framework for international health consultants*. Retrieved January 21, 2011, from www.whpa.org/pub2007_IHC.pdf

Wright, M. G. M., Zerbe, M., & Korniewicz, D. M. (2001). A critical-holistic analysis of nursing faculty and student interest in international health. *Journal of Nursing Education, 40*(5), 229–231.

Yang, Y. N., Xiao, L. D., Cheng, H. Y., Zhu, J. C., & Arbon, P. (2010). Chinese nurses' experience in the Wenchuan earthquake relief. *International Nursing Review, 57*(2), 217–223.

Zuyderduin, A., Obuni, J. D., & McQuide, P. A. (2010). Strengthening the Uganda nurses and midwives association for a motivated workforce. *International Nursing Review, 57*(4), 419–425.

APPENDIX A

CULTURAL COMPETENCY RESOURCES

Amerson, R. (2010). The impact of service-learning on cultural competence. *Nursing Education Perspectives, 31*(1), 18-22.

Andrews, M. M., & Boyle, J. S. (2007). *Transcultural concepts in nursing care* (5th ed.). Lippincott Williams & Wilkins.

Campinha-Bacote, J. (2011). The process of cultural competency in the delivery of health care services. Retrieved April 4, 2011, from www.transculturalcare.net/Cultural_Competence_Model.htm

Centers for Disease Control and Prevention (2011). Cultural competence. National Prevention Information Network. Retrieved April 4, 2011, from www.cdcnpin.org/scripts/population/culture.asp

Cross Cultural Health Care Program. (2011). Retrieved April 4, 2011, from http://www.xculture.org/

Ethnomed. (2011). Integrating cultural information into clinical practice. Retrieved April 3, 2011, from http://ethnomed.org/

Fadiman, A. (1997). *The spirit catches you and you fall down.* New York: Farrar, Straus and Giroux.

Galanti, G. (2008). *Caring for patients from different cultures* (4th ed.). Philadelphia, PA: University of Pennsylvania Press.

Giger, J. N., & Davidhizar, R. E. (2007). *Transcultural nursing: Assessment and intervention* (5th ed.). St. Louis: Mosby.

Hablamos Juntos. (2011). Improving patient provider communication for Latinos. Retrieved April 4, 2011, from http://www.hablamosjuntos.org/default.about.asp

Harrison, L. E., & Huntington, S. P. (2001). *Culture matters: How values shape human progress.* Basic Books.

Leininger, M. M., & McFarland, M. R. (2005). *Culture care diversity & universality: A worldwide nursing theory* (2nd ed.). Sudbury, MA: Jones and Bartlett.

Leininger, M. M., & McFarland, M. R. (2002). *Transcultural nursing: Concepts, theories, research and practice* (3rd ed.). McGraw-Hill Professional.

Lipson, J. G., & Dibble, S. L. (2005). *Culture & clinical care* (5th ed.). UCSF Nursing Press.

National Center for Cultural Competence (2011). *The mission of the NCCC.* Retrieved April 3, 2011 from http://nccc.georgetown.edu

Purnell, L., & Paulanka, B. (2008). *Transcultural health care: A culturally competent approach* (3rd ed.). F. A. Davis.

Spector, R. E. (2008). *Cultural diversity in health and illness* (7th ed.). Prentice Hall.

GLOBAL HEALTH AND MEDICAL RESOURCES

Bill and Melinda Gates Foundation. The foundation is focused upon building partnerships to save lives where help is needed most. Available at www.gatesfoundation.org/Pages/home.aspx

Birn, A., Pillay, Y., & Holtz, T. H. (2009). *Textbook of international health: Global health in a dynamic world* (3rd ed.). Oxford University Press USA. (Hardback available at www.amazon.com/exec/obidos/ISBN=0195300270/ladiesdrinkingso/)

Farmer, Paul. (2001). *Infections and inequalities: The modern plagues.* University of California Press. (Paperback, updated with a new preface, available at www.amazon.com/Infections-Inequalities-Plagues-Updated-preface/dp/0520229134/ref=pd_sim_b_1)

Farmer, Paul. (2003). *Pathologies of power: Health, human rights, and the new war on the poor.* University of California Press. (Hardcover)

Farmer, Paul. (2010). *Partner to the poor: A Paul Farmer reader* (California Series in Public Anthropology). H. Saussy (Ed.). University of California Press. (Paperback available www. amazon.com/Partner-Poor-Farmer-California-Anthropology/ dp/0520257138/ref=pd_sim_b_2)

Garrett, L. (2001). *Betrayal of trust: The collapse of global public health.* New York: Hyperion.

Global Alliance for Nursing and Midwifery Communities of Practice. The alliance creates opportunities for nurses and midwives to share knowledge and expertise to build capacity to improve health. Available at http://knowledge-gateway. org/ganm

Global Fund for Women. This organization is dedicated to promoting economic security, health, education, and leadership for women. Available at www.globalfundforwomen.org/ index.php

Global Health Council. The Global Health Council is a membership alliance dedicated to saving lives by improving health around the world. Available at www.globalhealth.org/

Global Health Delivery Online. Dedicated to improving health delivery through online collaboration. Available at www. ghdonline.org/

Global Health Education Consortium. This is a consortium dedicated to improving the ability of the global workforce to meet the needs of underserved populations. Available at http://globalhealtheducation.org/SitePages/Home.aspx

Global Health eLearning. Available at www.globalhealthlearning.org

Holtz, C. (2008). *Global health care: Issues and polices.* Sudbury, MA: Jones and Bartlett.

Jaret, P., Salmon, M., & Kasmauski, K. (2008). *Nurse: A world of care*. Atlanta, GA: Emory.

Kristof, N. D., & WuDunn, S. (2009). *Half the sky: Turning oppression into opportunity for women worldwide*. New York: Vintage.

Merson, M. H., Black, R. E., & Mills, A. J. (2005). *International public health: Diseases, systems and policies* (2nd ed.). Sudbury, MA: Jones & Bartlett.

O'Neil, E. (2006). *Awakening Hippocrates: A primer on health, poverty, and global service*. Chicago, IL: American Medical Association.

O'Neil, E. (2006). *A practical guide to global health service*. Chicago, IL: American Medical Association.

Skolnick, R. (2008). *Essentials of global health*. Sudbury, MA: Jones and Bartlett.

Unite for Sight. A non-profit global health delivery organization that empowers communities worldwide to improve eye health and eliminate preventable blindness. Available from www.uniteforsight.org

Weinstein, S. M., & Brooks, A. M. (2007). *Nursing without borders: Values, wisdom, success markers*. Indianapolis, IN: Sigma Theta Tau International.

World Health Organization. General resources. Available at www.who.int/en/

World Health Organization. International travel and health. Available at http://www.who.int/ith/en

Yong Kim, J., Millen, J. V., Irwin, A., & Gershman, J. (Eds.). (2002). *Dying for growth: Global inequality and the health of the poor*. Common Courage Press. (Paperback)

APPENDIX B

SELECT VOLUNTEER ORGANIZATIONS FOR NURSE VOLUNTEERS

AMERICAN COLLEGE OF NURSE-MIDWIVES

Silver Spring, Maryland, USA

www.midwife.org

Health professionals serve as consultants in programs around the globe. Nurse-midwives are given preference and consultants are paid. Service can be from 2 weeks to 3 years.

CAM INTERNATIONAL

Dallas, Texas, USA

www.caminternational.org

CAM International is a Christian missionary organization. Volunteers serve in Latin America. They offer some opportunities for health professionals.

CATHOLIC MEDICAL MISSION BOARD

New York, New York, USA

www.cmmb.org

Volunteers for Catholic Medical Missions Board (CMMB) must be licensed health care volunteers. Volunteers generally provide direct care to patients or provide medical training for local health care providers. CMMB offers both long-term and short-term assignments. Those who volunteer for 1 year or more receive reimbursement.

DOCTORS FOR GLOBAL HEALTH

Decatur, Georgia, USA

www.dghonline.org/

Doctors for Global Health (DGH) promotes health, education, art, and other human rights throughout the world. Volunteer nurses serve in inpatient and outpatient, community and public health settings. Average stay is about 3 months.

DOCTORS WITHOUT BORDERS (SEE ALSO MEDECINS SANS FRONTIERES)

New York, New York, USA

www.doctorswithoutborders.org

Volunteers must be licensed and have at least 2 years of professional experience. Volunteers might set up and staff clinics, work for public health campaigns, or serve in disaster areas. Commitment is usually 6 months to 1 year. Volunteers have all costs covered.

HAITIAN HEALTH FOUNDATION

Norwich, Connecticut, USA

www.haitianhealthfoundation.org/

Volunteers from the United States, Canada, and Europe travel to Haiti at their own expense to assist in the health programs in Jeremie, Haiti. Volunteer trips are usually about 1 week to 10 days in duration.

HEALTH VOLUNTEERS OVERSEAS

Washington, DC, USA

www.hvousa.org

Licensed health professionals serve in countries around the world. Nurses and nurse anesthetists from the United States and Canada have program partners. Volunteers serve as educators for the local health care professionals where they serve. Assignments are usually 1 month or longer. Volunteers cover their travel, but in many locations room is covered or offered at minimal cost.

MEDECINS SANS FRONTIERES (SEE ALSO DOCTORS WITHOUT BORDERS)

Headquarters in France, but volunteers come from all over the world

www.msf.org/msf/

Volunteers must be licensed and have at least 2 years of professional experience. Volunteers might set up and staff clinics, work for public health campaigns, or serve in disaster areas. Commitment is usually 6 months to 1 year. Volunteers have all costs covered.

OPERATION SMILE

Norfolk, Virginia, USA

www.operationsmile.org

Nurses and nurse anesthetists work with reconstructive surgical teams. Most volunteer missions are 2 weeks. Volunteers pay an organization fee, but travel and room and board are covered.

PARROQUIA SAN LUCAS TOLIMAN

New Ulm, Minnesota, USA

www.dnu.org/service/sanlucas.html

This is a program in Guatemala for education, housing, health, and agricultural development. Volunteer nurses and health professionals work in clinics. Most volunteers stay for 3 weeks. Volunteers do not receive a stipend.

PARTNERS IN DEVELOPMENT

Ipswich, Massachusetts, USA

http://www.pidonline.org/

Partners In Development (PID) works with families in Haiti and Guatemala to help them move forward from lives of poverty. Health volunteers work in PID's clinics in Port au Prince, Haiti, or in the Guatemala highlands. Volunteers stay in housing on-site but pay an organizational fee that covers housing and donation.

PARTNERS IN HEALTH

Boston, Massachusetts, USA

www.pih.org/

Partners In Health (PIH) does not generally send short-term volunteers to work in its projects overseas. However, the website shows a number of ways to become involved with its projects.

VOLUNTARY SERVICE OVERSEAS

Offices in Ottawa and Ontario, Canada, and London, United Kingdom

http://www.vsointernational.org

Voluntary Service Overseas (VSO) matches specific project needs with focused skills for the volunteer. Most assignments are for 2 years, and volunteers receive airfare and a living stipend.

APPENDIX C

GLOBAL HEALTH NURSING RESOURCES FOR FACULTY AND STUDENTS

This appendix lists examples of programs run by schools of nursing for undergraduate students, graduate students, or both.

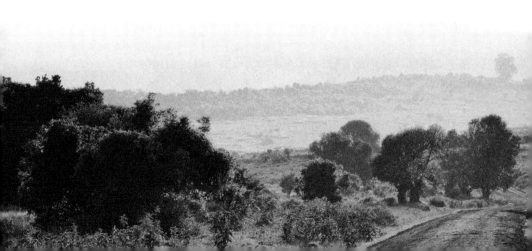

BOSTON COLLEGE
www.bc.edu/schools/son/aboutus/international/nicaragua/
background.html

BRIGHAM YOUNG UNIVERSITY GLOBAL HEALTH AND HUMAN DIVERSITY
http://nursing.byu.edu/global/default.aspx

EMORY UNIVERSITY
www.nursing.emory.edu/lccin/index.html

COLUMBIA UNIVERSITY
www.nursing.columbia.edu/globalHealth/index.html

CREIGHTON UNIVERSITY
www.creighton.edu/nursing/programs/mastersprogram/
mastersprogram/advancedpublichealthglobalhealthnursing/
index.php

DUKE UNIVERSITY
http://nursing.duke.edu/modules/son_global/index.php?id=15

EMORY UNIVERSITY
www.nursing.emory.edu/lccin/

GEORGETOWN UNIVERSITY
http://nhs.georgetown.edu/internationalhealth/learning/

INDIANA UNIVERSITY SCHOOL OF NURSING
http://nursing.iupui.edu/news/global_health.shtml

JOHNS HOPKINS UNIVERSITY
www.nursing.jhu.edu/, link to Areas of Excellence and then to Global Nursing

MCGILL UNIVERSITY
www.nusglobalhealth.webs.com/

NATIONAL UNIVERSITY OF IRELAND, GALWAY, IRELAND
www.nuigalway.ie/nursing-midwifery/Service%20Learning/

NSNA GLOBAL INITIATIVES IN NURSING COMMITTEE
www.nsna.org/ProgramActivities/GlobalNursing.aspx

SEATTLE UNIVERSITY
www.seattleu.edu/nursing/Inner.aspx?id=63050

UNIVERSITY OF ALABAMA
www.uab.edu/nursing/international-affairs

UNIVERSITY OF ARIZONA
www.globalhealth.arizona.edu/index.php?q=description

UNIVERSITY OF CALIFORNIA, SAN FRANCISCO
http://nurseweb.ucsf.edu/public/ing/

UNIVERSITY OF FLORIDA
www.nursing.ufl.edu/about_international_connections_ongoing_project.shtml

UNIVERSITY OF MARYLAND
http://medschool.umaryland.edu/ghrc/son.asp

http://nursing.umaryland.edu/collaborative-outreach/global-health-office

UNIVERSITY OF MIAMI
www.miami.edu/sonhs/index.php/sonhs/centers/pahowho_collaborating_center/exchange_programs/

UNIVERSITY OF MICHIGAN
www.nursing.umich.edu/global-outreach/going-global-students

UNIVERSITY OF MINNESOTA
www.sua.umn.edu/groups/directory/show.php?id=2231

UNIVERSITY OF NORTH CAROLINA
http://nursing.unc.edu/globalhealth/

UNIVERSITY OF PENNSYLVANIA
www.nursing.upenn.edu/gha/Pages/default.aspx

UNIVERSITY OF PITTSBURGH
www.globalhealth.pitt.edu/about/

UNIVERSITY OF UTAH
www.globalhealth.utah.edu/

UNIVERSITY OF VIRGINIA
www.nursing.virginia.edu/global/

UNIVERSITY OF WASHINGTON
http://nursing.uw.edu/academic-services/international-programs/
international-programs-at-the-school-of-nursing.html

UNIVERSITY OF WISCONSIN
www.son.wisc.edu/news/international.html

VILLANOVA
www.villanova.edu/nursing/global/

www.facebook.com/pages/Villanova-PA/Villanova-Nursing-
Global-Health-Experiences/108437807446

YALE UNIVERSITY
http://ysninternationalstudy.blogspot.com/

APPENDIX D

SERVICE LEARNING

In the following discussion, we briefly define various types of student learning for global health. In addition, we define service learning and give examples of service learning in nursing education and for global partnerships.

We define such faculty-student experiences according to 1) location, which is whether they occur at home or abroad; 2) purpose; and 3) characteristics. Nursing students learn about global health issues, nursing practice, and the global burden of disease in formal academic courses and through special informational programs at their school or college of nursing. Several colleges offer credit classes in international health or global health nursing.

GLOBAL HEALTH AT HOME

The American Association of Colleges of Nursing (AACN) notes in the *Essentials for Baccalaureate Education* that basic nursing education should include global health content (AACN, 2008). Schools and colleges demonstrate how this essential content is met in their own particular curriculum, so for some programs the essential content is incorporated into courses throughout the curriculum and in other programs. For example, the University of Pennsylvania School of Nursing offers a Multicultural/Global Health Care minor as part of its curricula options (http://www.nursing.upenn.edu/students/Minors/Pages/MulticulturalGlobalHealthCareMinor.aspx) as an elective, whereas at the Frances Payne Bolton School of Nursing at Case Western Reserve University, a required course called Health in the Global Community is a designated course (http://fpb.case.edu/courses/nurs.shtm). Many schools in the United States offer global health nursing as a certificate option or as an advanced practice educational focus. The London School of Hygiene and Tropical Medicine offers a certificate in Tropical Nursing. Examples of content from specialized courses includes cultural aspects of health care, the effect of socioeconomic and political factors on health and illness, the global burden of disease, health determinants, and the effect of policies to promote health globally.

INTERNATIONAL EXCHANGE PROGRAMS—LEARNING ONLY

Duffy, Farmer, Ravert, and Huittinen (2003) offer extensive information about an international exchange program between four universities in the United States and six universities in three European countries. Heuer, Bengiamin, and Downey

(2001) describe a faculty-led exchange program where students from the University of North Dakota travel to Russia. In addition, Ter Maten & Garcia-Maas (2009) report positive outcomes of role development for advanced nursing practice in an exchange program between nursing students at Rotterdam University and Texas Woman's University. In programs such as these, the goals focus directly upon the learner's needs, and neither faculty nor students provide a formal service to the host country. Though they build student knowledge about health care systems worldwide, generally they have no volunteer component, so we will not discuss these programs in depth.

SERVICE LEARNING

Service learning is a particular type of service and learning that meets clear criteria to advance service to community partners and mutual learning by academic and community partners. Peterson and Schaffer (1999) defined service learning as a "reciprocal relationship between students and communities in which both parties engage in service and learning" (p. 208). More recently service learning has been defined as "a teaching and learning approach that integrates community service with academic study to enrich learning, teach civic responsibility, and strengthen communities" (National Commission on Service Learning, 2009).

Key elements of service learning include the following:

- Reciprocal relationship between academic institution and community partners
- Clear connection to a course that allows for structured reflection and strategies to promote active learning and civic responsibility

- Opportunities for students to engage in structured reflection
- Learning activities to meet a community need
- Experiential learning
- Community being served controls the service provided

(Bailey, Carpenter, & Harrington, 2002; Indiana University Center for Innovative Teaching and Learning, n.d.; Sigma Theta Tau International Service Learning Task Force, 2009; Zlotkowski, 2007)

It is important to distinguish service learning from other forms of experiential learning. For learning to qualify as service learning, it must meet the specific requirements of a reciprocal relationship between academic and community partners to address a community need and offer opportunities for student reflection. Seifer and Vaughn (2002) emphasize that service learning is not synonymous with volunteering. Tied to curricula and community engagement, service learning must be sustained with institutional support. Bringle and Hatcher (1996) distinguish service learning from related learning or service initiatives such as community service, philanthropy, experiential learning, and pre-professional training experiences. For nursing, student clinical practicum experiences would be an example of the latter.

SERVICE LEARNING IN NURSING EDUCATION

Service learning in nursing education increases engagement with community members that strengthens students' knowledge of the context of health, health determinants, and population health (Drevdahl, Dorcy, & Grevstad, 2001;

Nokes, Nickitas, Keida, & Neville, 2005; Peterson & Schaffer, 1999). Examples from the United States represent the majority of nursing education examples (Bentley & Ellison, 2005; Gerberich, 2000; Hamner, Wilder, & Byrd, 2007; Reising, Allen, & Hall, 2006; Sigma Theta Tau International Service Learning Task Force, 2009), but other countries also report service learning programs (Casey & Murphy, 2008; Downes, Murray, & Brownsberger, 2007).

Seifer and Vaughn (2002) published a bibliography of service learning programs that includes projects with various groups in communities, such as older adults living in high-rise apartments, homeless persons, children in Head Start programs, and school children.

One published example of a global health service learning student experience is the Sister City Partnership between Indiana University School of Nursing and Posoltega, Nicaragua. "Student-learning activities included the following: developing relationships with community residents, providing prenatal classes, supporting nursing scholarships, and participating as interdisciplinary, multicultural team members" (Riner & Becklenberg, 2001, p. 234).

In another example, more than 2,200 nursing and other health professional students in universities in Ethiopia were sent to drought-stricken regions of Ethiopia. In their work they provided direct clinical care to patients, addressed nutritional needs, participated in preventive activities such as sanitation campaigns, and helped to train local professionals and others in the stricken regions (Downes, Murray, & Brownsberger, 2007).

In Chapter 6 we commented that currently there are neither standards for global health experiences for nursing students nor clear outcome expectations. In an effort to develop best practice principles for global service learning, McKinnon and Fealy (2011) offer seven core principles for developing global service-learning programs in nursing. We encourage faculty to critically analyze our global health educational programs to create ethical, responsible, partnered and mutually beneficial programs for students and host partners.

REFERENCES

AACN. (2008). *Essentials for baccalaureate education.* American Association of Colleges of Nursing.

Bailey, P. A., Carpenter, D. R., & Harrington, P. (2002). Theoretical foundations of service-learning in nursing education. *Journal of Nursing Education, 4*(10), 433–436.

Bentley, R., & Ellison, K. J. (2005). Impact of service learning projects on nursing students. *Nursing Education Perspectives, 26*(5), 287–290.

Bringle, R. G., & Hatcher, J. A. (1996). Implementing service learning in higher education. *Journal of Higher Education, 67*(2), 221–239.

Casey, D., & Murphy, K. (2008). Irish nursing students' experiences of service learning. *Nursing and Health Services, 10*(4), 306–311.

Downes, E. A., Murray, J. P., & Brownsberger, S. L. (2007). The use of service-learning in drought response by universities in Ethiopia. *Nursing Outlook, 55*(5), 224–231.

Drevdahl, D., Dorcy, K. S., & Grevstad, L. (2001). Integrating principles of community-centered practice in a community health nursing practicum. *Nurse Educator, 26*(5), 234–239.

Duffy, M. E., Farmer, S., Ravert, P., & Huittinen, L. (2003). Institutional issues and the implementation of an international student exchange program. *Journal of Nursing Education, 42*(9), 399-405.

Gerberich, S. S. (2000). Care of homeless men in the community. *Holistic Nursing Practice*, *14*(2), 21–28.

Hamner, J. B., Wilder, B., & Byrd, L. (2007). Lessons learned: Integrating service learning community-based partnership into the curriculum. *Nursing Outlook*, *55*(2), 106–110.

Heuer, L., Bengiamin, M. I., & Downey, V. W. (2001). The impact of international cultural experience on previously held stereotypes by American student nurses. *Multicultural Education*, *9*(1), 26–29.

Indiana University Center for Innovative Teaching and Learning. (n.d.). *Important documents for faculty*. Retrieved April 4, 2011, from http://citl.indiana.edu/ programs/serviceLearning/importantDocumentsFaculty.php

McKinnon, T., & Fealy, G. (2011) Core principles for developing global service-learning programs in nursing. *Nursing Education Perspectives*, *32*(2), 95–101.

National Commission on Service Learning. (2009). National service learning partnership. Retrieved April 4, 2011 at http://www.service-learningpartnership.org/site/ PageServer?pagename=sl_natlcommission

Nokes, K. M., Nickitas, D. M., Keida, R., & Neville, S. (2005). Does service learning increase cultural competency, critical thinking, and civic engagement? *Journal of Nursing Education*, *44*(2), 65–70.

Peterson, S. J., & Schaffer, M. J. (1999). Service-learning: A strategy to develop group collaboration and research skills. *Journal of Nursing Education*, *38*(5), 208–216.

Reising, D. L., Allen, P. N., & Hall, S. G. (2006). Student and community outcomes in service learning: Part 2-Community outcomes. *Journal of Nursing Education*, *45*(12), 516–518.

Riner, M. E., & Becklenberg, A. (2001). Partnering with a sister city organization for an international service-learning experience. *Journal of Transcultural Nursing*, *12*(3), 234–240.

Seifer, S. D., & Vaughn, R. L. (2002). Partners in caring and community: Service learning in nursing education. *Journal of Nursing Education, 41*(10), 431–439.

Sigma Theta Tau International Service Learning Task Force. (2009). *Service learning: Pedagogy of civic engagement for nursing.* Unpublished manuscript.

Ter Maten, A., & Garcia-Maas, L. (2009). Dutch advanced nursing practice students: Role development through international short-term immersion. *Journal of Nursing Education, 48*(4), 226–231.

Zlotkowski, E. (2007). The case for service learning. In L. McIlraith & I. MacLabhrainn (Eds.). *Higher education and civic engagement: International perspectives* (pp. 37-52). Ashgate, England: Aldershot.

INDEX

A